Pearls and Pitfalls in Forensic Pathology

Infant and Child Death Investigation

Pearls and Pitfalls in Forensic Pathology

Infant and Child Death Investigation

Darin P. Trelka
Forensic Pathologist
Assistant Professor of Clinical Biomedical Science and Director of Anatomical Programs at Florida Atlantic University, Boca Raton, FL, USA

Peter M. Cummings
Forensic Pathologist
Neuropathologist
Assistant Professor of Anatomy and Neurobiology, Boston University School of Medicine, MA, USA
Chief Medical Officer and CEO of Northeast Neuropathology and Autopsy Services, LLC, Boston, MA, USA

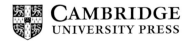

CAMBRIDGE
UNIVERSITY PRESS

CAMBRIDGE
UNIVERSITY PRESS

University Printing House, Cambridge CB2 8BS, United Kingdom

Cambridge University Press is part of the University of Cambridge.

It furthers the University's mission by disseminating knowledge in the pursuit of education, learning and research at the highest international levels of excellence.

www.cambridge.org
Information on this title: www.cambridge.org/9781316601525

First published 2016

Printed in the United Kingdom by Clays, St Ives plc

A catalog record for this publication is available from the British Library

Library of Congress Cataloging in Publication data
Names: Cummings, Peter M., 1971– , author. | Trelka, Darin P., author.
Title: Pearls and pitfalls in forensic pathology : infant and child death investigation / Peter M. Cummings, Darin P. Trelka.
Description: Cambridge ; New York : Cambridge University Press, 2016. | Includes bibliographical references and index.
Identifiers: LCCN 2015046423| ISBN 9781107040403 (hardback) | ISBN 9781316601525 (mixed media) | ISBN 9781139628945 (online)
Subjects: | MESH: Death | Forensic Pathology – organization & administration | Child | Infant Death | Cause of Death | Data Collection – methods | Documentation – methods
Classification: LCC RA1063.4 | NLM W 800 | DDC 614/.1 – dc23
LC record available at http://lccn.loc.gov/2015046423

ISBN 978-1-316-60152-5 Mixed Media
ISBN 978-1-107-04040-3 Hardback
ISBN 978-1-139-62894-5 Cambridge Books Online

Additional resources for this publication at www.cambridge.org/9781316601525

. . . .

We dedicate this book to our mentors and to all of those who will succeed us. For the latter, we hope this book helps to prepare and center you for this most arduous journey.

Contents

Preface

We hope that this text is used as a helpful guide through the business of death investigation.

As in all professions, initially there is a very steep learning curve, but this profession is, indeed, a bit different. When considering these dedicated men and women, never forget that of all the people in the world, *few are qualified or would even be capable* of performing the tasks of the death investigator. Because the crux of this profession is death and the determination of its causes and circumstances, the subject matter, while already complex, is made even more difficult in having to integrate the emotions of the families', loved ones', and significant others' witnesses (and even one's own) into the tragic work of the day.

The conversational writing style is intended to personalize the information in a more easily understood and memorable manner, just as if the reader were spending a day on scene or in the morgue with the writers. We hope that this text will extend the training of death investigators (i.e., medicolegal death investigators, coroners, medical examiners, forensic pathologists, forensic laboratorians, and law enforcement) and attorneys beyond the basic concepts learned in their standard training courses.

The text is centered in updated, practice-based, and hard-earned information on approaches to death investigation in order to clarify misunderstandings and to supplement training gaps. In addition, we have imparted personal experiences regarding death investigation as to policy, procedure, standards, and the anticipation of problems during death investigations. Interspersed throughout the text are procedural standards from the National Association of Medical Examiners and the Centers for Disease Control and Prevention, as well as effective administrative and management strategies for offices involved with death investigations. The ultimate goal of this text is for the reader to be able to use the information gleaned from the text for immediate and direct application to their casework the minute they put the book down.

Knowing that training in death investigation can be markedly non-uniform, it is our sincere hope that this text will both guide neophytes through their preparative and formative stages and also act as a referent for those who are in the process of gaining the myriad experiences needed for this truly Herculean undertaking. Know that training is truly never finished and that there is *always* something to learn from a death scene investigation.

Death investigators are most definitely a special lot and we wish you great success in all your endeavors. Good luck, be safe, and be great!

Darin P. Trelka, M.D., Ph.D.
Coconut Creek, FL

The birth of a textbook is often the result of frustration: frustration with the lack of resources or the lack of a cohesive resource tying all the tidbits of information together. Medical education is an apprenticeship where the young physician learns by listening to elders. Although this has been the tradition in medicine for centuries, this approach leaves gaps in information and produces information that is scattered throughout various resources. It was this feeling of frustration of not being able to find information that gave birth to our first textbook, *Atlas of Forensic Histopathology*, and to this most current effort, *Pearls and Pitfalls in Forensic Pathology: Infant and Child Death Investigation*. This new book is filled with, as I like to refer to, "things I wish I'd known then and things experience has taught me." There are plenty of excellent pediatric autopsy textbooks in the world but, as is often the case, the pathology is the least complicated component of a pediatric death investigation – you will see an obvious lethal injury, you will have findings on histology or in the laboratory studies. But what happens when the autopsy findings are completely negative? At this point you are left with the facts of the investigation – the investigation is your history. Above and beyond all else, I am a physician and the history of the patient is where the differential diagnoses are generated. The complexity of pediatric death cases rests in deciding how the autopsy results fit with a story; it could be the medical story (AKA the history) or the story given by caregivers. Whatever the situation, there are times when the point of the autopsy is to corroborate or refute a story. Being able to suss out that story is the point of this book. The autopsy is a single piece of information and it must be interpreted in the context of everything else known about the case. One does not make conclusions at the autopsy table, one makes observations and those observations are later formed into conclusions once all the information is gathered. Our new book will help the reader deal with the important non-pathology related aspects of a pediatric death investigation and serve as a guide of what to do from the moment the phone rings to report the death to the final signature on the death certificate. It is a manual for investigators, whether they are police, lawyers, medical examiners, coroners, or medicolegal investigators, which provides a logical approach to the investigation so that no information (or as little as possible) is missed. Basically, it is a reference on how to take a history. It has been said in the past that the most important tools for use by a forensic pathologist are a quiet room and a comfortable chair. In that regard, it is our hope that this text provides a scaffolding for the reader to organize their thoughts so that he or she can spend the necessary time to think as they work on these difficult cases.

Peter Cummings, M.Sc., M.D.
Boston, MA

Acknowledgments

Cases

Renee Robinson, M.D., Forensic Pathologist/Deputy Coroner, Stark County Coroner's Office, Canton, OH.

David M. Posey, M.D., Glenoaks Pathology Medical Group, La Cañada, CA.

Anna McDonald, Forensic Pathologist, Pediatric Pathologist, Assistant Professor, Wake Forest Baptist Medical Center, Winston-Salem, NC.

Death certification

Stephen J. Cina, M.D., Chief Medical Examiner, Cook County Medical Examiners Office, Chicago, IL.

Background and setting of death investigation

Introduction

Medicolegal death investigation is a team sport with shared, complementary duties to be performed by multiple professionals. It begins with the discovery of the dead body, before the arrival of the first responders, and continues until the certification of the death and court adjudication. Every piece of it from beginning to end is important to resolve as completely as can be, and all parts must make sense to the investigator(s) involved. Ignoring even one detail, however small and seemingly unimportant, can lead to the lack of resolution of case elements and misinterpretation of data. All deaths are based in context, and it is this context that will lend the most assistance in proper certification of each death case. The professionals on the team must be able to convey their interpretation of data as well as be able to incorporate the expertise that other teammates bring to the case. Very importantly, all players must know their own role and, in well-constructed death investigation systems, should understand how they fit into the larger picture. The perception that the medical examiner or coroner "will figure it out at the autopsy" is thankfully becoming extinct. In fact, what should be stressed is that the autopsy findings are merely one set of data among a backdrop of *many* other pieces of information, which have to be examined and resolved for any of the findings to make sense.

The perspectives have changed over the last few years and newer ideas and more well-defined systems are being synthesized under various and sundry "selective pressures." In addition, it cannot be underscored enough there is *not one model to fit every jurisdiction*, thus it is important to realize that not every jurisdiction will do things in the same way. Although it would be ideal to try to unify procedures and policies, idiosyncratic properties such as proper staffing; differential training and experience of death investigators, medical examiners, coroners, forensic pathologists, law enforcement, and attorneys; interest (or lack thereof) by the overseeing government; and the availability of resources *really* steer the process. It is the combination of these "selective pressures" that sets the tone for the commencement of death investigation in these systems. The main idea of this book and of death investigation in general is that, above all else, deaths have to be investigated fully from the outset, because once information is lost or forgotten, it is often gone for good. A final consideration is that of the concept of assumption. Assumption in any investigatory endeavor, be it death investigation or survey of French literature, is the bane of that endeavor. Anyone can *assume* information, in that it does not require a shred of training or expertise. The point of true investigation is to clarify information as much as it can be clarified under the circumstances of the case, and be able to draw lines of linkage between events in the chronology of the cases. If there is a question to be asked…ask it. If there is information that is required to understand a particular set of data, acquire that information. An oft-spoken adage is that "if you don't look, you'll never find," and this defines effective investigation.

Death investigation

First, it is important to point out and understand that medicolegal death investigation and criminal investigation are *two separate entities*, though they often intersect at the point of a decedent (i.e., dead body) and the associated scene. Law enforcement is concerned with criminal investigation and is usually focused on whether a crime was committed and, if so, identifying potential suspects and witnesses. The focus of death investigation, alternatively, is the determination of how the person came to be dead (i.e., cause of death), the circumstances (manner) of the death (i.e., homicide, suicide, accident, or natural), and what information at the scene, imparted by witnesses, in the first responder records, or the medical records can help determine the cause, and manner, of death. The duties within death investigations are usually separated and organized by statute and credentialing, but the systems must work in concert if the case is to be resolved appropriately.

The primary roles of the medicolegal death investigation system are to determine *cause* and *manner* of death for deaths in which the city, county, or state jurisdiction has been established through statute. Jurisdictional criteria for death cases are usually very similar across all geographical areas, but do demonstrate state- or county-based historical idiosyncrasies. In short, jurisdiction is established in deaths that are:

1. Violent (i.e., homicidal, suicidal, and/or accidental in nature)
2. Suspicious
3. Unexpected (i.e., when in previously good health or in childhood)
4. As a result of intoxication or poisoning
5. Unattended (defined by statute or administrative order of the jurisdiction)
6. As a result of employment
7. When in some form of incarceration
8. When a result of undiagnosed disease as a potential threat to public health.

Therefore any deaths that are reported to the death investigation system and reach the threshold, by circumstances of the aforementioned criteria, are "accepted" and will be investigated by various modalities such as records review, external examination, or autopsy. Alternatively, those cases that do not reach jurisdictional criteria are "turned down." In the United States, death investigations are undertaken and certified by either a coroner or a medical examiner. The coroner system dates back to feudal Europe and, as such, is the oldest death investigation system in existence.

Coroners are elected officials who, depending on the state, may or may not be a physician, can sometimes be a forensic pathologist, but may also be a layperson with no training in death investigation or forensics, whatsoever.

Medical examiners are physicians (by definition) who are appointed by political figures and who are usually under the auspices of a forensic pathologist Chief Medical Examiner, board-certified in *at least* anatomic and forensic pathology by the American Board of Pathology (ABP).

As stated, the death investigation system has two roles: the determination of *cause* and *manner* of death. To define terms, "cause of death" is the disease, the injury, or the poison, which creates the anatomic or physiologic insult culminating in death. This is considered the empirical (observational) or "scientific" part of the investigation. Commonly accepted examples of causes of death are hypertensive and arteriosclerotic cardiovascular disease, gunshot wound of the head, and acute cocaine intoxication. The task of cause determination is completed via several different means, including external physical examination, performance of an autopsy, or through collection and careful review of voluminous medical records based on clinical assessment(s) of the decedent and their state(s) of health.

The "manner of death," is defined as an *opinion* of "what happened" to the decedent (i.e., homicide, suicide, accident, or natural), and is based upon the circumstances derived from scene analysis, witness accounts, and investigation by the medical examiner/coroner and law enforcement. Manner determination has very little to do with the external or internal examination of the body, although the anatomic findings can be *consistent* with a particular manner of death. For example, a contact gunshot wound of the head *is consistent* with a suicide, but could also be a homicide if the witness or forensic evidence suggests it to be so. Multiple gunshot wounds to the head from any muzzle-to-target distance, or intermediate- or distant (indeterminate)-range gunshot wounds are *generally inconsistent* with a suicidal manner. *Manner of death is not determined by autopsy; rather, manner of death is determined by thorough investigation of the known circumstances and placing the findings of autopsy into the context established by those circumstances.* It is analogous to, and an extension of, the practice of medicine in that a regime of treatment is almost never based on a single physical examination or laboratory-based datum of a patient. In most cases, proper treatment is based in the context established by a thorough history of present illness, medical history, surgical history, allergies, family history, psychosocial history, review of systems, physical examination, laboratory studies, and imaging studies as appropriate. Once all these parts have been dissected and salient facts elucidated, a defensible list of differential diagnoses can be generated, further studies can be entertained in order to further resolve the elements of the differential diagnoses, and any treatment initiated will usually be far more effective and clinically specific.

The death investigation system: a primer

Medicolegal death investigators, autopsy technicians, photographers, forensic pathologists, odontologists, anthropologists, entomologists, toxicologists, and forensic scientists are the "players" in the modern death investigation system (excluding law enforcement and the system of *juris prudence*, which is beyond the scope of this book), and they must integrate their disciplines in order to properly certify these deaths. At the core of the effective medicolegal death investigation system lies a competent and well-trained staff of investigators. For the purposes of this book, the term death investigator is inclusive of all personnel involved in death investigation and includes medicolegal death investigators, medical examiners, coroners, forensic pathologists, laboratory personnel, and law enforcement. In certain cases, first responders (i.e., fire rescue, fire fighters, and paramedics) and even clinicians can also be considered "death investigators" and are important parts of the death investigation system.

Investigations

Investigative personnel must be available 24 hours a day, 7 days a week not only to answer initial "death calls," but also to respond to death scenes; to take jurisdiction over the bodies; to make decisions on injury patterns; to resolve, identify, and collect evidence for receipt to law enforcement; to begin identification procedures where indicated; and to assist in analysis of the scene as the context in which the death occurred. These investigators should have specialized training in death investigation, should be able to effectively and independently triage trauma versus natural disease, be familiar with medical language and its connotations, and be certified by the American Board of Medicolegal Death Investigators (ABMDI).

Pathology

The pathology department often has two arms: one described as the autopsy technician or "pathologist's assistant," and the other filled by the physician forensic pathologist. The duty of the pathology department is to perform autopsies or external examinations on decedents to determine the absence or presence of an anatomic cause of death. At the exclusion of, or to clarify the importance of an anatomic cause, pathologists must collect tissues and fluids for laboratory study in order to determine an infectious, physiologic, or toxicologic cause. In addition, the pathology department has the duty to collect evidence from without and within the bodies for submission to forensic laboratories.

Consultative laboratory services

Death investigation systems (as well as law enforcement agencies) also employ innumerable laboratory scientists: the toxicologists who process, identify, and quantify the soluble toxicants in the body fluids submitted from autopsy and external examinations; forensic scientists who are the specialists of trace evidence, toolmarks/firearms, questioned documents, fingerprints, and blood spatter, who collect, process, and visualize the trace evidence from the scenes and decedents to establish the inextricable linkages between them. Finally, there are the molecular biologists who process the fluids and tissues from scenes, bodies, evidence, and clothing in order to establish biologic identification to ascertain and demonstrate the genetic unity required between defendant(s), victim(s), and the scene.

Photography and digital imaging

Photography, photo documentation, and image processing are crucial requirements for medicolegal death investigation and have been since the nineteenth century. Proper visual documentation of death scenes, the decedent, and all of the trace evidence therein is of paramount importance before any physical assessment of the body is made. Photography is not only used for documentation purposes during acquisition of trace evidence from the body, but also is important during the autopsy as a visual record of injuries, natural diseases, wound patterns/sizes, and to assist in the demonstration of wound directionality when indicated. In fact, when properly executed, many argue that the entire autopsy can, and should, be able to be recreated photographically for any medical or legal official, or, in criminal cases, for the judge and jury. The photographer must not only be well trained in standard camera function/operation, but also all autopsy dissections and techniques used to demonstrate trauma, natural disease, and all related anatomic relationships with regard to what they typically demonstrate and what images should be captured. Digital imaging specialists have facility with the myriad techniques needed to visualize objects of interest, such as the use of alternative light sources, variable light angulation to resolve complex patterns, film speeds and exposure times, the use of color correction to impart the image as it was captured in the autopsy suite or on scene, and knowledge of the ever-expanding armamentarium of digital technology, image-enhancement software, and new imaging techniques. It has also become crucial that the modern medicolegal death photographer capture the initial images in a format that is legally, and universally, recognized as not having not been modified or enhanced in any way.

Forensic odontologists

Forensic odontologists, or dentists, have two main roles, which are to assist in the identification of as yet unknown decedents through charting of the teeth of decedents and comparison with exemplar antemortem dental charts, as well as to assess patterned injuries that may have resulted from a human (or non-human animal) bite.

Forensic anthropologists

Forensic anthropologists can assist in identification of unknown skeletal remains by determining gender, age, height, and race, as well as examining the skeleton for stigmata of disease processes and for the discrimination of antemortem injuries from postmortem changes (taphonomy).

Forensic entomologists

Forensic entomologists analyze insect species associated with dead bodies in order to determine time since death and possibilities of whether the body may have been moved after death or where the body may have been stored or secreted after death.

Support staff

Finally, in the modern medical examiner/coroner's office, there are the support staff whose importance cannot be numerated and whose contributions are legion. These are the people who process the paperwork, transcribe the dictations, and experience the illness, violence, and death of the subjects of the office through the written and spoken record(s) of the various death investigations and reports they handle. There can be no measure of their value (despite how the governmental management and budget "sees" and reckons their importance), or the infinite support exhibited by these people in the face of monumental tragedy, the likes of which governmental benefactors and most of the general public cannot begin to fathom. These staff members must "push the paper," create the networks, fix the software, and streamline the perpetual flow of death though the office, all without any medical training or hazard pay, and with acceptance that their job is never complete, for the dead will always keep coming.

For these hard-working staff, there is only the satisfaction borne of the knowledge that they alone, often personally, assure the families of decedents that all that can be, has been done, that the cases will be expedited to the best of the office's ability, and that nobody will forget the sacrifice(s) made by the decedent and the families.

Pivotal role in education of community

In the face of the voluminous day-to-day work of the office, many medical, scientific, and investigatory staff also engage in education through both informal tutorial at the laboratory bench/autopsy table as well as more formalized teaching via academic appointments in local universities, through recognition at professional conferences, and through peer-reviewed research. There is near-constant didactic, practical, and small group-based "teaching" of medical, allied health, law enforcement, and legal authorities with regard to the daily findings of the casework. Above and beyond that, it is common that medical examiner/coroner's staff will even appear in local secondary schools, hospitals, and police/fire stations in order to lecture on forensic science to both educate and inform. In fact, major changes in departmental policies and procedures for all agencies related or involved with death investigation (i.e., law enforcement, hospitals, fire-rescue, etc.) can be discussed, codified, and implemented in this fashion. These contributions are often made on personal time and without any financial remuneration. It is the cause of many offices and practitioners not only to be competent specialists in their various professions, but also to "take the word out" to all those who would hear it.

In summary, today, the local medical examiner- or coroner-based medicolegal death investigation system is more than just an office that processes "bothersome" dead bodies or for performance of free autopsies that hospital pathologists no longer feel qualified or comfortable performing, regardless of what role it may have played historically in its jurisdiction. The value of the office also has nothing to do with the sum total number of cases it processes, as in an office that processes 8,000 decedents must be "better" than one that processes 1,000; rather, its value is most appreciated for the number of death investigations it investigates *to completion*. As such, the staff of these institutions have to have the financial *and* political support of the local government and their chief medical examiner or coroner. These talents are not inexpensive, they do not "come cheap," and as such are often the culmination of years of expensive education, trials, and tribulation: a fact that cannot be ignored by employers or by the financial officers of the jurisdiction(s). The staff of these offices cannot be equated with any other county or state workers (despite the degree to which this is illogically attempted by governmental administrators), must be appropriately compensated for their level of achievement, the sacrifices they have made, and those they continue to make for their continued competence in their respective fields. In addition, the staff should be financially and philosophically supported in their continued education and maintenance of their various certifications. It is the only true way to ensure that the positions will be held by highly qualified people who will use accepted, gold-standard procedures in order to competently process their casework. This means not only having monies available for meetings and training, but also enough staff to cover the work of the day while new staff are being trained. These staff not only have to perform to excellence every day, but they also must be able to recruit trainees to their offices and training programs to be educated and properly instructed and nurtured, ensuring a renewable supply of well-qualified forensic scientists.

The death investigation system stands as a sentinel, a beacon, which alone can speak for the dead and stands to help to ensure justice for all involved. These offices have all of the characteristics of a physician's office, hospital-based clinic, reference laboratory, and academic institution complete with students, trainees, and faculty members. These attributes, difficult for any one entity alone to practice well, must be balanced carefully and carried out while still functioning under the auspices of the local government with all of its limitations and idiosyncrasies. The need for understanding and philosophical congruence between the offices and their governmental supporters should be sought after above all else if the office is to carry out the duties with which it has been charged. These duties are completed through various means such as numerous educational benefits to the community at large, excellent medicolegal consultation, constant technological maintenance and improvement, and a complete and thorough final report of investigation, which is assembled from the work products of all of the staff of the office. It is all of these things, done every day, which become the measurable quantity of its worth.

Death investigation is a holistic art and cannot be practiced in a vacuum. It demands the cooperation of all practitioners and the need for agreement between the anatomic findings, investigation, and scene elements. Each datum must be interpreted within the context of the scene and investigative findings, and should never be overinterpreted. The case in its final form with cause and manner of death is a *mosaic* of the findings and interpretation(s) of many death investigators with varied experiences and skill sets. All players must know their duties and what they have to do. In addition, all players should be interested in *streamlining*, *updating*, and *validating* their processes. An efficient death investigation system is seamless in its workings, they have reduced redundancy, practice gold-standard forensic procedures, and all players understand their role(s) as they relate to their jobs and interpretations of the other players.

History and philosophical issues

History

The history of infant and child death investigation has been reviewed recently (Collins and Byard, 2014) and the discussion of the dispersion of myth and pseudoscience in this venture has been thoroughly documented. What is important to understand with regard to death in the young is that infants and children have different sensitivities to insults (up to a point) than adults and these sensitivities are based, in part, on the idiosyncrasies of their relatively unique anatomy and physiology, which have been reported in great detail elsewhere. That having been said, in the business of death investigation, nothing takes the place of being thorough, a good set of eyes, solid training, and an inquisitive mind. It cannot be overstated, in fact, the importance of the inquisitive mind as it drives forward the wont of the investigator to answer questions to satisfaction and completion. In any death investigation, regardless of the age of the decedent, the investigator must not stop asking questions until they are satisfied with the answers given with regard to the consistency of that information with the physical findings of the scene and decedent. There will be numerous people in various fields of interest (law enforcement, attorneys, families, other death investigators) who will attempt to reduce the amount of work that they are forced to do, who will do the least amount of work they can in any situation, who will accept the easy or most simplistic explanations in order to try to boost their closed case list, or who will make linkages between likely unrelated things and occurrences in order to make cases appear more straightforward. The death investigator must stand firm and rely on science, empiricism, experience, and logic to guide them in their quest for information. If the case information is not making sense, the death investigator must decide what data they will have to see, read, or hear, which will satisfy their questions; and if that is either not possible or is not made

available to them, the death investigators have the option of certifying either cause or manner of death as "undetermined" because they do not *have* the information required to discriminate between causes or manners within a reasonable degree of medical certainty. Along the same lines, it must be remembered that the certification of cause and manner can be amended if additional, probative information becomes available, which changes the mind of the certifier. In fact, this very statement is a good idea to have in the opinion section of the autopsy report following the signature of the certifying physician. It enables the reader to understand that no case is actually "closed" and that a case may be amended.

It was not so long ago that some forensic pathologists, medical examiners, and coroners thought, or were trained to believe, that they could answer all of the questions regarding a death strictly from their examination of the body during autopsy. Following evidence-based practices and the principles employed in clinical medicine, subsequently the tide has thankfully turned away from this archaic and potentially dangerous practice in favor of gathering all of the material information as early as possible. Modern death investigators are properly trained and sanctioned by a governing body and feel comfortable going to death scenes and investigating deaths in parallel with law enforcement. Well-trained death investigators realize the power of observing the body in the context of the death scene and are able to relate scene elements to the body in order to assist in pattern recognition and to help direct law enforcement inquiries *at the scene*. The American Board of Medicolegal Death Investigators (ABMDI) provide the gold standard training modality for death investigators and it should be the goal of every medical examiner/coroner's office to be fully staffed with board-certified medicolegal death investigators. Pathologists in training, colloquially known as "fellows," are also being trained in this approach to death investigation and this writer has found great success with approaching cases in this manner, rather than accepting another person's assessment of the scene. In fact, since forensic pathologists perform the autopsy, which means to "see for oneself," intensive training regarding visiting the scene with the body in place to help interpret findings on, or in, the body by scene examination, and even following body removal as they convey the body to the morgue, have been important pieces to understand in the overall death investigative "puzzle." The forensic pathologist in training should understand all of the processes of the death investigation from the first death call to decision making about scene visitation, to visiting the scene, interacting with all of the players at the scene, proper scene visitation etiquette, the vagaries of evidence acquisition and transfer to law enforcement personnel, chain of custody, when to call for body removal, and proper transportation of the decedents. By doing so, any hindrances or issues that develop in the process (and, believe me, they will) can be mitigated with minimal impact on case certification.

Philosophy behind infant and child death investigation

While we like to believe that death will never come to the young, it unfortunately does. Those deaths that are patently due to clinically well-documented natural causes (i.e., metabolic disorders, anatomic aberrations, infections, etc.) are generally excluded from medicolegal investigation, as when properly investigated and triaged they do not generally meet jurisdictional criteria for acceptance and have typically been followed closely by a treating physician who will certify the death as natural. Those child deaths that *do* appear to be violent or unexpected/unnatural (i.e., when in apparent good health and with no compelling antecedent medical history to which to ascribe cause of death) will naturally fall under the acceptance jurisdiction of the death investigation system. Some of the deaths that fall under medical examiner/coroner jurisdiction will be of occult natural disease processes, some will be accidental in nature and resulting from motor vehicle crashes, injuries while at play, entrapment in household apparati,

choking, inadvertent ingestion of intoxicating substances, and drowning, and yet others will be due to inflicted insults such as blunt or sharp-force injuries, gunshot wounds, non-accidental asphyxia, volitional starvation by caregiver(s), or other form of neglect, and poisoning. There are a group of deaths in childhood and infancy in which the cause of death will be undetermined, wherein no anatomic, physiologic, or chemical basis for death will be elucidated and in which case scene findings are unrevealing. In these undetermined deaths, subsets will be due to all the aforementioned etiologies, but are unable to be demonstrated with a reasonable degree of medical certainty. In these cases, it is generally best, at least for the sensibilities of the authors, to certify the deaths as undetermined and to explain to the family and other officials the demonstrable findings, the lack of compelling lethal findings, potentialities for cause of death, and the limitations of the autopsy and postmortem laboratory testing process.

In consideration of the aforementioned generalities, stratifying the deaths into age groups is an efficient and meaningful way to consider and discuss these deaths and death investigation.

Infant death

Infancy is conventionally defined as the first year of life. Deaths during infancy can be stratified into three general categories. The first is natural, due to congenital anatomic malformations, metabolic disorders, or infections, which commonly occur, especially in the first month of life. The second category is trauma, which can be further split into accidental (non-inflicted) and non-accidental (inflicted) trauma. The third is the general category of sudden unexplained infant deaths (SUID), which is a "waste basket" certification and includes deaths due to unclear means including what was formerly known as sudden infant death syndrome (SIDS).

Traumatic deaths in infancy can happen during any period within the first year of life, albeit a thankfully rare occurrence. With regard to forensic medicine, the most important consideration in traumatic infant death is whether it can be considered accidental or non-accidental. For some of these confusing cases where trauma may have played a role in the death of an infant, a good rule of thumb is that any lethal injury in a child under the age of one year, which results or can be implicated in death, should be investigated as a homicide *until proven otherwise*.

Why think of these deaths in those terms?

It is conventional that infants are well protected, are almost constantly in the company of adult caregivers, and by the virtue of their immature neuromuscular status, are unable to engage in any "high speed," "great height," or "risk-taking" behavior, which is unlike that seen in older children and adolescents. Using that logic, cases of violent deaths in infants will begin to resolve themselves quickly into those wherein infants have died (1) in motor vehicle crashes or under other like unfortunate traumatic circumstances, which are witnessed and explainable; (2) those deaths that are clearly due to *inflicted* injury; and (3) those few cases that can be considered "in between" in which manner would be certified as undetermined.

As unwitnessed and as yet unexplained, the latter two categories of cases must be investigated fully, including interview of all people involved (i.e., caregivers, family members, etc.) or anyone who may have knowledge of the circumstances; interview of medical staff who have treated the decedent (if the decedent was treated in a medical facility); careful review and objective interpretation of medical records in cases where the infants are taken to the hospital; and performance of an autopsy with full toxicology and employment of metabolic and microbiologic assays (where indicated).

In doing all these things, one can (1) document and categorize the acute injuries; (2) establish the existence or absence of any natural disease states that may explain or even mimic injury(ies) (yes, they can and do); (3) check for remote injuries in order to establish the existence or absence of a "pattern of injury" consistent with remote or chronic abuse (i.e., comminuted rib fractures, fractures on contralateral sides of the body, fractures of various ages that have no logical or documented traumatic etiology, or remnants of hemorrhage around or within the brain or within the body cavities); and (4) permit time for a proper investigation by child protective services (as warranted), law enforcement, and the medicolegal death investigation system. The number, type, severity, and complexity of the injuries must be considered and correlated with the known and reported circumstances in order to determine temporal reasonability.

As an example, consider a three-month-old infant who is admitted to the hospital with a closed head injury including *complex* right temporo-parietal skull fractures, scalp contusions on the right *and left* sides of the head, and intracranial hemorrhages, whose caregiver states that the infant "fell in the bathtub" during a bath while the mother was at work. This particular story is one commonly associated with and reported in the context of infant head injuries, and the death investigators must *immediately* reckon its inconsistency with regard to the chronological age and abilities of the child and with the spectrum of injuries. The head injuries in this example are very severe, and are clearly outside the spectrum, type, quality, and severity typically seen in common household injuries sustained by an infant. Secondly, an important question to be answered is why are there injuries on *both* sides of the head?

A simple fall, or even a surreptitious drop, of the infant may include one impact site of the scalp, but why on *both* sides in this example? This raises the question of at least two spatially separated head impacts, which are inconsistent with a simple fall or drop. Another important concept is that of developmental milestones of infancy and childhood and using these as a context within which to assess the caregiver's report of events (see Table 2.1).

Thus by being aware of normal developmental milestones, a death investigator would know that a three-month-old infant would not developmentally be able to stand in the bathtub in order to "fall." An infant of that age would not likely even be able to support themselves with their arms yet, certainly not yet able to crawl, so a "fall" in the tub would be virtually impossible in this example.

In this case, there must be another explanation for the injuries and this should be conveyed to law enforcement so that a more directed set of questions can be asked of the caregiver, armed now with the context of the spectrum of injuries. In addition, the circumstances can be rendered even more questionable if there has been documentation of previous injurious episodes of the same child, or previous children in the same household, or in the presence of the same caregiver. The presence of healed or healing injuries, or previous medical documentation of trauma can help to better define this unlikely pattern of injuries in an infant.

These are not binary decisions, meaning it is not, "if this or these types of injuries, then abuse." One must consider all facets of the case to determine the likelihood or inconsistency of its elements and, as such, may

Table 2.1 Developmental milestones

Age	Social and emotional	Language communication	Cognitive	Movement and physical development
2 months	• Begins to smile • Briefly calms self • Tries to look at parent	• Coos, gurgling sounds • Turns head towards sound	• Pays attention to faces • Recognizes people from distance and follows with eyes • Acts bored (cries, fussy)	• Smoother movements with limbs • Able to hold head up • May push up when on stomach
4 months	• Smiles spontaneously • Likes to play with others, cries if stops • Mimics facial expressions	• Babbling sounds with expressions • Different cries with different needs (hunger, pain)	• Expresses happy or sad emotions • Reaches for objects (toy) with one hand • Beginning of hand/eye coordination • Watches faces closely • Follows moving things with eyes	• Head is steady, without support • Pushes legs down when feet are on a surface • Possibly able to roll over from stomach to back • Can hold toy and shake it • Hands to mouth
6 months	• Starts to recognize familiar faces • Knows if someone is a stranger • Likes to look at self in mirror • Likes to play with others, especially parents	• Makes sound in response to other sounds • Responds to name • Makes sounds to express happiness/discomfort	• Looks around at nearby things • Tries to get to things out of reach because of curiosity • Passes things back and forth between hands	• Rolls over in both directions • May be able to sit without support • Rocks back and forth • Might crawl backwards before moving forwards
9 months	• Fearful of strangers • May be clingy with familiar adults • Develops favorite toy/object	• Understands "no" • Sounds may resemble words • Points at things • Copies sounds	• Plays peek-a-boo • Picks up tiny things (cereal) between index finger and thumb • Looks for things that are hidden	• Stands with support • Crawls • Able to get into sitting position without support • Pulls to stand up
12 months	• Cries when parents leave • May assist with dressing/care	• Responds to spoken requests • Uses simple gestures • Few basic words • Tries to repeat spoken words	• Shakes, bangs, throws things out of curiosity • Finds hidden items easily • Able to point out correct object when you name it • Uses brush, cup, other objects correctly	• Uses furniture to cruise • May take a few steps without holding on • May be able to stand without assistance

Adapted from Centers for Disease Control and Prevention Developmental Milestones (www.cdc.gov/ncbddd/actearly/milestones/index.html) with permission from the CDC.

take a considerable amount of time in order to determine the veracity of the circumstances.

Sudden infant death syndrome and sudden unexplained (or unexpected) infant death

Sudden unexplained (or unexpected) infant death (SUID), a descriptor utilized by the Centers for Disease Control and Prevention (CDC), pertains to those infant deaths that are unexplained, such as what was previously known as sudden infant death syndrome (SIDS) (Figure 2.1).

What you will note from the website is that the CDC is evidently still unclear as to what this entity is and what it should be called. Thus, if the cause of death is undetermined due to negative anatomic, laboratory, or scene findings, then the manner must be undetermined, and until or unless more probative information is brought to light, it remains undetermined … a far more honest approach to this human-mediated nomenclature issue.

The typical case of undetermined death (which used to be certified as SIDS or SUID) is one where a four-month-old infant has been having cold symptoms

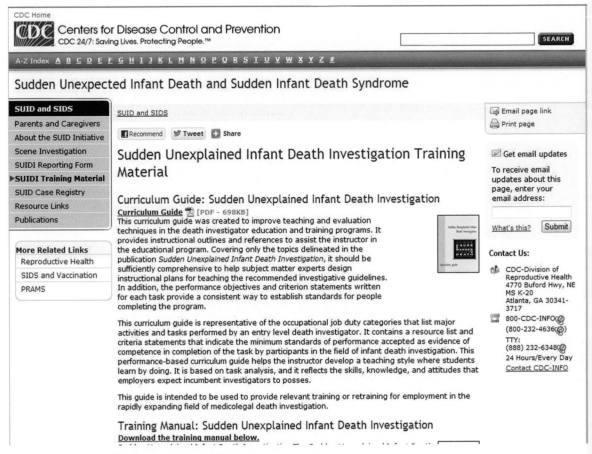

Figure 2.1 Screen capture from the Centers for Disease Control and Prevention website, reproduced with permission from the CDC. If you note the discrepancy between "sudden unexplained" and "sudden unexpected" infant death, the issue becomes that those who have interest have promulgated SUID as a certification for "the sudden unexpected death of an infant under one year of age while in apparent good health whose death may have been a result of natural or unnatural causes," which means that since no one expects a car crash, infection, a metabolic aberration, anatomic malformation, and/or for a caregiver to abuse an infant, SUID could be certified in place of "multiple blunt force injuries," bacterial meningitis, congenital hypothyroidism, truncus arteriosus, or the typical heretofore employed construct known as "SIDS," which are undetermined for cause and manner of death. Much confusion has come out of this as one can imagine and any epidemiologic statistics based on death certification as SIDS, SUID, or undetermined certifications will be difficult, if not impossible, to interpret.

for the last couple of days, was fed and placed down to sleep in a crib. Three hours later the caregiver checks on the infant to find him unresponsive in the crib. Emergency medical services (EMS) are called and they will usually convey the infant to the hospital despite the lack of any vital signs. To enable the use of a certification of undetermined, in lieu of the aforementioned SIDS or SUID, certain criteria must be fulfilled. The infant must have a full autopsy with full toxicology, microbiological testing (such as blood, spleen, lung, and cerebral spinal fluid cultures, where indicated), and a nucleic acid panel for inborn errors of metabolism (if the state panel has not been performed).

Thus, for cause (and thus manner) of death to be considered undetermined, all of these assays, laboratory tests, and examinations (both gross and microscopic) must be negative. In addition, the forensic pathologist must review medical records including birth records and the state metabolic panel, pediatrician records, records from any hospitalizations, and, if any, the fire rescue and hospital record of the death.

In addition, as soon as is possible after finding the dead infant, a reconstruction of the death should be performed in the residence with the caregivers and law enforcement personnel present and engaged. After the lack of positive anatomic and laboratory findings, the cause of death still cannot be certified as undetermined unless the reconstruction is also negative, meaning there cannot be any indication of suffocation with the infant face down on a non-breathable sleep surface, positional or mechanical asphyxia with the infant wedged between the bed and the wall, or being found unresponsive underneath an adult while co-sleeping.

Philosophical parameters in certifying these deaths are as follows. If the autopsy and laboratory findings are negative, the past medical history is benign, and the scene reconstruction demonstrates the infant was placed face up in a "naked crib" (i.e., no blankets, no extraneous bedding, toys, or other materials that can possibly asphyxiate the infant), the death can be considered for a certification of undetermined. Cause of death being undetermined, therefore, means that after thorough investigation (including anatomic, laboratory, and scene examination), a cause of death is not able to be determined to a reasonable degree of medical certainty.

There are infants who die of, as yet, unknown phenomena – and this certification permits recognition of that. There is a growing movement of forensic pathologists who will certify the cause of death in these cases "undetermined," rather than giving the certification a relatively meaningless name and creating a mystique that SIDS or SUID means "something," rather than, in fact, meaning "nothing."

If almost all the criteria previously mentioned are fulfilled – with the exception of scene elements, which remain as concerning – or if the scene reconstruction cannot, or will not, be completed, the cause of death should also be considered for certification as "undetermined," which is defensible as there are elements of the case that are either worrisome or unknown, and it is forensically prudent to recognize the gaps in the data and certify the death conservatively and without bias. In these cases the certification can both be explained verbally to the family or caregivers, and also be elaborated upon in the opinion section that each autopsy report should have.

Deaths in childhood and adolescence

As children become more mature, they have less sensitivity to environmental perturbations, they are more skeletally and muscularly robust, their nervous system matures to one accustomed to terrestrial life at normal Earth gravity, and their physiology is successively more in line with established adult parameters. Death investigations during this maturation period also fall more in line with those utilized for adult deaths. Compulsory scene reconstructions become less import, because children and teenagers can self-extricate from potentially lethal positional trauma and thus asphyxia due to co-sleeping becomes a non-issue. The causes of death are still relative in distribution, though the number and types of natural diseases shift into another range as do the number and types of traumatic causes of death, which become more numerous and varied if only because children and adolescents become spatially separate from parental protection as they begin ambulating, riding, sledding, swimming, jumping, rolling, playing, driving, and being driven. In addition, as children get older, recreational drug use becomes an item on the list of differential diagnoses, which only ascends in importance into adulthood. It is also in this group that death investigators must take care to collect thorough historical information (both medical and social) as there can be traumatic sequelae from events during birth and infancy that cause long periods of morbidity and, if not contextually organized, appear to be potentially natural to the uninitiated. The jurisdictional magnitude will often become clear when asking the correct questions during triage and subsequent interview of the death reporter.

System diversity and jurisdictional items

Training and expertise: diversity is good

The forensic pathologist is a medical doctor, a physician, who has successfully completed four years of medical school (either allopathic or osteopathic), three to four years of pathology residency (anatomic pathology, or combined anatomic and clinical pathology, respectively), and at least a one year of forensic pathology fellowship for their specialized training. Because the practice of medicine, and forensic medicine is indeed included, is relatively idiosyncratic, and is based in each practitioner's academic background, medical school education, life experience, residency training, and clinical experiences, very few forensic pathologists are "the same" in their approach to medicolegal cases, though many of the processes are conventionally (thankfully so) universal.

In previous years there were many pathologists who called themselves "forensic" pathologists who had no specialized training, and who may never have been certified by the American Board of Pathology in anatomic, clinical, or forensic pathology. Because of their lack of specialized training, the validity of their findings and their opinions were potentially questionable and were often not held in check by quality control measures or oversight by a Board-certified forensic pathologist. Most recently, and completely appropriately, there has been a movement by the forensic pathology governing body, the National Association of Medical Examiners (NAME), to assure that for certification by their governing body, offices are staffed by Board-certified pathologists who have the specialized training and experience required for this profession. This is not to say that there have not been, or are currently not, some absolutely outstanding forensic pathologists who have successfully completed their forensic fellowships, but have not achieved certification by the American Board of Pathology. It is likewise

ridiculous to consider that Board certification somehow imbues upon its diplomates all knowledge about the field. However, Board certification does show that at least during the time they passed their Board examinations that they had some objectively documented degree of mastery of the material. In any event, in this day and age and under the ever-mutable machinations of the legal system, it is forensically prudent that pathologists who are performing forensic autopsies should either be certified in forensic pathology or at least be overseen by a Board-certified forensic pathologist.

As alluded to earlier, there are many ways, means, and mechanisms to practice forensic pathology, although there are some guiding principles that have been discussed. There are offices that have a jurisdiction so geographically widespread that scene visitation is all but impossible. There are jurisdictions where there are such operational and philosophical rifts between law enforcement and the medical examiner/coroner that death investigators are purposefully not informed of deaths, that scenes are not maintained or kept intact for death investigators, or that death investigatory staff and forensic pathologists are explicitly unwelcome at death scenes, despite any extant statutory provisions.

There are some medical examiner/coroner offices that have historically performed death investigations by request of families or other interested parties because the medical examiner or coroner believes that as tax payers, the requests of the public should be universally honored. There are offices where differing levels of toxicologic inquiry are performed on *every* case, despite the logic (or lack thereof) of the policy, and regardless of the cost, the investigational findings, external examination or autopsy status, or autopsy findings. There are other offices where toxicology is performed only when there is investigational reason or when there is no appreciable gross or microscopic anatomic cause of death. There are offices where they have done away with their "in-house" toxicology laboratory as a cost-saving measure such that all of their testing is sent out to a local reference laboratory as needed. There are offices that are directly associated with their own crime laboratory and have forensic scientists on staff and available for consultation or assistance at a moment's notice, and yet other offices where they are so isolated from law enforcement and the local county or state crime lab that they have no idea how particular results may have affected the case or the ascertainment of injuries on the decedent. There are offices where the coronership has been granted to political figures or law enforcement despite the clear perception of the conflict(s) of interest that this arrangement may represent. There are offices where the coroner must statutorily be a physician, and others where the coroner is a layperson with no training in death investigation or death certification practices. There are offices where every scene is visited by a forensic pathologist, and other offices that employ forensic pathologists who have little to no death-scene experience. There are offices where forensic pathologists perform the autopsies, but the coroner or chief medical examiner adjudicates the cause and manner of death, and yet others where the forensic pathologists actually run the day-to-day functions of the office and the coroner or chief medical examiner is only there very peripherally to follow the progress of casework and to collect materials for their next government appointment. There are offices where decisions about autopsy or external examination are made by state attorneys rather than the decision being made by trained forensic pathologists or physician medical examiners. There are offices that cover so large a jurisdictional area that several offices must be strategically geographically placed in order to efficiently serve the needs, and within these, local physician medical examiners or "field MEs" make jurisdictional decisions as well as investigational decisions, such as case requirement for external examination or autopsy. There are offices where forensic pathologists may perform over 400 complete autopsies a year and other offices where the forensic pathologists have *never* gotten above 200 autopsies a year (including externals, which NAME counts as a third or a fifth of a complete autopsy). There are offices in which the forensic pathologists do everything including scene examination, evidence collection, photography, radiological services, dental charting and identification, and their own forensic

anthropology – with very little assistance by subject matter experts or even clerical staff, which is in contradistinction to offices where forensic pathologists almost never even touch the bodies in favor of permitting forensic technicians, pathologists' assistants, or "dieners" to perform the bulk of the actual dissection and evisceration. There are offices that have fleets of well-trained and Board-certified medicolegal death investigators on 24 hours a day, 7 days a week; other offices that have only a secretary to triage cases and make case decisions; and yet other offices where the forensic pathologist, medical examiner, or coroner are taxed with triaging every death call and scene request. There are offices that are staffed by forensic pathologists who can perform six to ten autopsies a day, all by themselves with no assistance, and offices in which there is a cut off of two to three examinations a day in favor of pathologists not being physically overworked. Furthermore, there are permutations of all the above with mixtures of medical examiner and coroner systems within the same jurisdiction or a mosaic medical examiner/coroner system within the same state.

In consideration of the myriad approaches to death investigation, there are forensic pathology fellowship training programs associated with many of these permutations and, as such, there are multiple ways that trainees are taught to practice and function, though all have to conform, in function and spirit, with the Accreditation Council for Graduate Medical Education (ACGME) and the standards set forth by NAME. It is because of this diversity of performance and function that there are innumerable ways to approach forensic cases – and one of the reasons a book like this is so very important in the understanding of the death investigation system in the United States.

The depth and variability of training ensure a richness and diversity that permits these offices to function, sometimes in spite of themselves and in spite of, at times and in some cases, morally despicable supportive neglect by the state and local governments, local law enforcement, local legal systems, and their associated administrators. There are certain offices that will never be funded to the level they should because of administrative failures on both sides of the political "podium," but the offices are still statutorily charged with carrying out their functions…thus the forensic pathologists have to learn how to do as much as they can (within legal, moral, and professional limitations) in order to be effective agents for their discipline and for their constituents. In contrast, there are offices that have not only a rich historical tapestry, but also access to expertise and equipment that permit their staff and trainees to carry out "cutting edge" death investigations, that many in the field can only familiarize themselves with through reading the literature. Though certainly arguable, it is conceptually important for practitioners of death investigation to move around enough not only to spread their gifts and experiences, but also to continue to learn techniques and ways of handling situations with which they would never have been presented had they stayed in one spot. Additionally, being witness to different policies and procedures makes the practitioner knowledgeable about what works and about how to see to the efficient completion of the workload in various offices with differing levels of support. Also, having worked in numerous offices enables the practitioner to realize when the political and philosophical opposition to efficiency and case completion is too great to be overcome – and thus to know when to vacate those positions.

It is this diversity of education, training, and background that enriches the offices and helps to maintain a semblance of professional evolution. It permits the spread of good ideas and practices, enables other practitioners to see and experience what you bring to the office, and ultimately serves the forward movement of the profession as a whole.

Jurisdiction

Death investigators, be they forensic pathologists, lay-physician medical examiners, coroners, medicolegal death investigators, or laboratorians, investigate deaths under the legal authority of the office with which they are associated (Clark *et al.*, 1996). The authority of the office is based in the state, county, or local laws/codes that govern the role(s) of the medical examiner/coroner (Clark *et al.*, 1996). Thus it is important that the first thing that staff in the medical examiner/coroner role do is to familiarize themselves with the applicable statutes and administrative codes as the parameters within which they can and must operate. In addition, familiarity with the applicable statutes/administrative code will not only guide decision making in difficult cases, but will also enable the death investigation system to explain pertinent legal parameters to inquiring families, law enforcement, and legal officials.

The death investigation system should be in constant contact with the Office of Vital Statistics of that town or county in order to be facile with information regarding death certificates, as well as the often chaotic business of burial, cremation, and transport of decedents (Clark *et al.*, 1996).

The applicable statutes and administrative codes will generally contain information regarding which deaths are reportable, who may report death, who may pronounce death, who has jurisdiction over the dead body, the role of law enforcement in assisting with investigation, who is responsible for identification of the decedent, the determination of next of kin or "legally authorized person," who may receive the decedent's personal effects and valuables, what defines an unclaimed body, who notifies the next of kin or "legally authorized person" of the death, whether an autopsy can be performed without the consent of the next of kin or "legally authorized person," the process of the family requests for no autopsy on the basis of personal or religious beliefs, and the time period of notification of law enforcement of the death (Clark *et al.*, 1996).

The death investigators should also be familiar (both professionally and procedurally) with other agencies with which they interact: such as district, state, or Commonwealth attorney's office; infant death working group(s); Occupational Health and Safety Administration (OSHA); local health department; local adult or child protective service(s); National Transportation and Safety Board (NTSB); and local law enforcement agencies (i.e., federal, state, county, and city).

It cannot be overstated that the medical examiner/coroner's office must work within the parameters set by statute and code – with no deviation or purposeful ignorance of these directives. Statute and code serve to (1) guide decisions; (2) direct not only medical examiner/coroner staff but also *all* other agencies as to their role(s) in death investigation; (3) define the role of the office in the jurisdiction where it exists; as well as (4) *protect* the office and its staff when making decisions that are religiously, culturally, emotionally, or politically unpopular with its end users (i.e., families of decedents, law enforcement, attorneys, healthcare providers, and religious groups). It is a relatively common occurrence that a decision or directive of the medical examiner/coroner's office is questioned or countered by various end users and being facile with, and in agreement with, statute and code will inform the protestors and help keep the offices procedurally, legally, and philosophically on track.

For example, when faced with a family- or legally-authorized person who does not want their loved one's body to be transported to the medical examiner/coroner's office for external examination or autopsy, it is completely appropriate to mention to the protestor that they are asking the office to break the law and that the statute or code is clear on what defines jurisdictional criteria and the process of death investigation. Death investigators can guide protestors to the appropriate section of the statute or code, or can even send them web links to the same. Many jurisdictions have the latitude to permit the family to seek judicial interdiction if they wish to stop an examination or autopsy where the medical examiner/coroner has full authority (by statute or code) to make whatever examinations they deem necessary to adjudicate cause and manner of death. In these cases, a reasonable time frame should be given to the family or their representative (i.e., 48 to 72 hours) and if the judge orders the medical examiner/coroner's office not to perform said examinations, then it is that judicial authority which will rule and the medical examiner/coroner's office will appropriately concede responsibility to the judge. Thankfully, this is a rare occurrence, but being aware of how to handle these cases is crucial to efficient operation, as they come up periodically. If there are any questions about statute or code or how to approach these issues, the state, county, or city attorney associated with the medical examiner/coroner's office (all of them are associated with a guiding attorney in some fashion) should be consulted and a legally consonant course of action should be taken.

What cases to report

In general, most jurisdictions are guided by statute or code to determine the cause and manner of death, and are generally empowered to make or have performed such examinations, investigations, and testing as is seen fit by the medical examiner/coroner, or as requested by the state attorney when any person dies in the state/county:

1. of criminal, accidental, or suicidal violence
2. in any circumstance suspicious for criminal, accidental, or suicidal violence
3. suddenly, when in apparent good health
4. unattended by a practicing physician (will have a time frame defining time period of being unattended)

5. in police custody (to include all penal institutions or during arrest)
6. by criminal abortion
7. by poison or other intoxicating substance(s)
8. by disease constituting a threat to the public health
9. by any employment-related disease, injury, or toxicity
10. when dead bodies are brought into the jurisdiction with inappropriate medical certification
11. when a body is to be cremated or buried at sea
12. unidentified remains.

Again, these are generalities and the specific statutes and codes guiding offices must be known by staff of those offices. Using these rules, the office will understand the types of cases that should be reported to them, and know which they will accept under these criteria and which they can refuse.

Types of cases typical for infant and child death investigation include clandestine feti, deaths on scene, and hospital deaths.

Clandestine feti

The first example of typical cases that come to the attention of the medical examiner/coroner are deaths wherein feti have been found surreptitiously hidden in garbage cans or dumpsters, wrapped in plastic bags or newspapers, or just left in an out-of-the-way location and found by a passer-by. Occasionally these decedents will be found mummified or skeletonized and buried in backyards or tucked away in shoeboxes and placed in wall constructions or under floorboards. In any case, the first question from law enforcement is always the cause of death and close in chronology will be the question of whether the infant was born alive. As a corollary to the latter question is the ascertainment of the infant's developmental age. This is important because if the infant is less than 22 to 23 weeks of gestation, there is no extra-uterine survivability. Thus there are many questions to be answered in these cases relatively quickly. Law enforcement may wish to know to whom the fetus belongs, which is nearly impossible to tell without a reference sample from the suspected mother. There are criteria for live birth listed in the literature; however, only food (i.e., breast milk or formula) in the gastric contents is defensible anatomic proof of a period of viability. If there is any degree of

15

decomposition at all and no evidence of food in the stomach, it is very difficult to determine a period of postpartum viability. A commonly quoted test from the older literature described the placing of a piece of liver and a piece of lung into cups of water in tandem. The reported interpretation of the results was that: (1) if both the liver and lung pieces sink, then the infant never took a breath; (2) if the liver sinks and the lung floats, then the infant took a breath; and (3) if the lung and liver both float, then there is likely to be some decomposition and formation of gas from bacterial metabolism. The interpretation of the results of the aforementioned "test" is difficult due to so many mitigating uncontrolled circumstances (i.e., if upon birth of a "dead infant" where the mother attempts even one rescue breath by blowing into the infant's nose, mouth, or both, this scenario could artificially inflate the lungs and give the appearance that the infant had taken a breath, were the aforementioned "test" utilized in this case). Thus interpretation of this test is difficult, at best, and the results can be indefensible. In these cases, the infant should be taken back to the morgue and morphometric measurements taken and compared to conventionally accepted charts in order to determine an approximate gestational age. If the gestational age is determined to be above the limit of viability (i.e., 22 to 23 weeks), then it is *possible* that the infant had some period of viability. Unless there is other proof of postuterine life (i.e., witnessed movement, crying, milk in the gastrointestinal tract, etc.) not much may be able to be said other than the baby "may have been born alive."

Deaths on scene

Infant deaths at home where the body is still at the scene may be a rarity in some jurisidictions. Rescue units seem to tend to transport infants to the nearest hospital *pro forma*, despite clear evidence of lack of life signs, but this likely depends on the area, the policies of the first responder unit(s), and their level(s) of training. The typical scene is one where an infant has been found dead on a sleep surface of some kind (i.e., bassinette, crib, couch, in bed with caregivers, or in bed with siblings or other relatives). The body has usually been moved because of the panicked life-saving efforts and the general mobility of the decedent in the hands of a frantic parent. Upon arrival of the death investigator or forensic pathologist, the infant is usually face up and demonstrates the

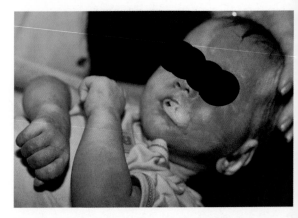

Figure 3.1a Deceased infant with foam emanating from the mouth and patterned, fixed livor mortis on the anterolateral (left) side of the face. Note the geographic area of pallor on the right side of the face and alternating areas of pallor and livor on the left side of the scalp and left earlobe. The infant was reportedly found in a head-in-declination position with the head trapped between the crib railing and the crib mattress. The livor and pallor patterns are consistent with that historical datum.

stigmata of attempted resuscitative efforts. The caregivers are almost never in the residence at that time as they are either being consoled or interviewed by law enforcement, which permits the examination of the decedent. Following the investigators being updated about the reported circumstances from law enforcement, the infant will be photographed and externally examined. Examination and correlation of the pattern (if present) of livor mortis can give an indication as to the positioning of the decedent when found (Figure 3.1a and b).

Note if the caregiver's narrative of the finding of the baby is inconsistent with the physical findings upon examination of the body (i.e., livor patterns that are inconsistent with the reported position of the body when found) such that, as in this example, if the caregiver reported that the infant was found lying supine in the crib with a blanket up to its abdomen, it is clear by the livor and pallor patterns on the head of the decedent that the infant's head was *between* two objects after death as there are the aforementioned geographic pallor on the right side of the head and the alternating areas of fixed livor and pallor on the left side of the head. Thus the physical findings would be inconsistent with the reported story. At this point in the example, the death investigator can demonstrate to law enforcement the physical findings and the caregiver(s) can be re-interviewed armed with the external examination findings in order to clarify the positioning of the infant

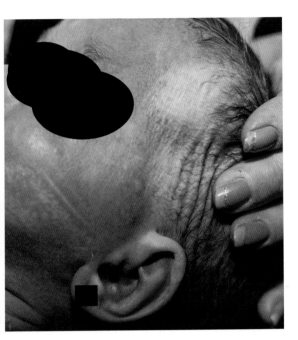

Figure 3.1b Closer photograph of the alternating areas of fixed livor and pallor on the left side of the scalp as well as on the convex surfaces of the left earlobe.

who last saw the infant alive and who found the infant (if they are separate people) should be interviewed by the death investigator/forensic pathologist in the presence of law enforcement. This permits the death investigator/forensic pathologist the opportunity to hear the events directly from the witnesses and also serves as a control for the consistency of the stories imparted by the witnesses. It is at this time that a scene reconstruction can be scheduled, the earlier the better, while all the materials associated with the infant death (i.e., blankets, sleep surface, witnesses, bottles, toys, paraphernalia, etc.) are available in nearly an "as is" state (see Infant death scene reconstruction).

As discussed, deaths in older children are generally handled similarly to those of adults as they are less sensitive to benign environmental insults.

Hospital deaths

Hospital deaths usually require no visitation unless the infant or child was brought to the hospital acutely unresponsive and was pronounced dead upon arrival. In these cases, it may be important to visualize the decedent, be able to document a body temperature, and to confirm what, if any, laboratory tests were drawn and sent for assay. Appearance of the death investigator or forensic pathologist at the hospital for deaths following admissions of any significant length are of nearly no value as there is no scene to appreciate.

right there at the scene. In addition, the place the infant was found can be examined and correlated with the findings from examination of the body. If there are no findings suspicious for inflicted injury, the caregiver(s)

The death call

Death call

Medicolegal death investigators are charged with documenting every call they receive regarding deaths in their jurisdiction. The vast majority of the reported deaths will be natural, but each should be handled and investigated in order to understand the nature of the death within a reasonable degree of medical certainty (Clark *et al.*, 1996). Death calls that are reported to the office are documented based on office policy and procedure, but generally they are of two varieties: those in which the cause and manner are natural (i.e., colloquially "turn downs" or "non-ME cases") and those that reach jurisdictional acceptance criteria (i.e., colloquially "ME" or "coroner" cases).

The medicolegal investigator must collect various pieces of information (some of which are conventional and some of which are based in the office policy and procedure) and this information is usually contained within standardized forms that will eventually be included for review or in the case file.

The reporter of death will, in the vast majority of cases, be a member of law enforcement (i.e., either a road patrol officer or a homicide detective) who is calling from the scene, or a physician, nurse, or decedent affairs specialist from a hospital.

Citizen report of death

If a citizen or civilian (i.e., not a healthcare official or member of law enforcement personnel) is calling the office to report a death, it is appropriate and encouraged to first take their name, location (i.e., theirs and the decedent's), and if that is unknown, any visible or nearby architectural or geographic landmarks, the caller's contact information, the identity of the decedent (if known), and then to direct the caller to call the local 911 dispatcher to report the death to law enforcement. Once the telephone call is finished, it is advisable and encouraged for the death investigator to immediately place a call to the appropriate local law enforcement agency and report the death yourself so that law enforcement and fire rescue are made aware of the call just received and to give them the opportunity to respond to the scene in case the citizen reporter decides not to follow up as directed.

The majority of medical examiner/coroner offices are not directly associated with law enforcement agencies and, as such, have no arrest or criminal investigative powers. Thus law enforcement must, and should be, the first responders to a death scene outside a hospital. The reporter may be considered a suspect until proven otherwise and having law enforcement be able to interview the reporter may be critical in the case.

Considering the above example, the death report may be erroneous, and the subject may actually be unconscious, but still alive, and law enforcement and fire rescue as first responders may save that life. In addition, medical examiner/coroner offices have jurisdiction over *deaths* only, thus if the subject is still alive, medical examiner/coroner staff have no legal authority to be involved in the case. Finally, without any consideration or knowledge of the location or circumstances of death, it is not forensically prudent that medical examiner/coroner staff respond to what may be a crime scene without law enforcement first investigating the circumstances, and examination and documentation of the scene.

Law enforcement death calls

The information generally to be collected is as follows (Clark *et al.*, 1996):

1. Date and time of the report.
2. Name and official title of the reporter, including agency name, badge number (if law enforcement), and all relevant contact numbers.

3. Reason and circumstances under which the death is being reported (i.e., died at home, motor vehicle crash, homicidal violence, death in a hospital, etc.).

4. Decedent demographic data (i.e., name, sex, race, birth date, address, social security number, marital status, phone numbers, identification status and identified by whom, next of kin or legally authorized person, and the location, date, and time of death notification of same, employment history, etc.).

5. Death event data (i.e., location, date, and time of death pronouncement; location, date, and time of being last seen alive and by whom; location, date, and time of any injury to the decedent, etc.).

6. Decedent medical history (i.e., recent complaints [if it is a verbal child or adolescent], to whom they were made and under what circumstances; history of the pregnancy [if an infant]; birth history [if an infant or young child]; name of primary care physician and any specialists the decedent have seen; medical conditions for which the decedent was being treated; prescribed medications [if any]; when the decedent was last seen by their physician and why; any hospitalizations).

7. Circumstances of death (i.e., *chronological* narrative of the known recent events in the decedent's life to include any pertinent remote history, the recent past prior to having been found dead, the circumstances of finding the decedent [location, time, by whom, why was the finder present, etc.], and what has occurred since the death was recognized, who reported the death, etc.).

8. Discovery of death (date, time, location found; position when found; ambient temperature, presence of clothing [as appropriate]).

9. Any previous acute life-threatening events (ALTE) (i.e., cardiorespiratory arrests, asthmatic issues, fainting, suicide ideation or attempts, etc.).

10. Any previous police involvement at this address, or between the cohabitators of the decedent or involving the decedent.

11. Any medications, illegal drugs, or drug paraphernalia present.

12. Any involvement by other agencies (i.e., adult or child protective services, hospice, visiting nurse, etc.).
(Adapted from Clark *et al.*, 1996)

The cases that do not reach jurisdictional criteria are usually logged and are to be reviewed by the medical examiner or coroner as a measure of quality control in order to assure the correct jurisdictional decision was made. Those cases that reach jurisdictional criteria are then further investigated and a decision must be made to visit the scene or not, and the decedent will eventually be either transported to the office for examination or held at a hospital or funeral home for examination, depending on the jurisdiction and its policies and procedures.

Scene visitation: to go or not to go?

In general, scene visitations are always educational and bring a level of understanding of the case that even the best verbal narratives never seem to capture. The bulk of the important information one needs to know to resolve the case is found at the scene with the body in place. In fact, an argument can be made that the vast majority of the information for effective death certification is sought from initial scene examination and when correlated with anatomic and positional findings on the body, that subsequent external examination and autopsy are only to verify the items on your list of differential causes. The death scene is as important as the examination of the body and, in some cases, is the crux of the death case. For example, in cases of positional or mechanical asphyxia, there may be few or no "specific" anatomic findings on the body and the autopsy and toxicology may be completely negative. The prudent death investigator, where either a scene visit was unavailable or if the body was moved prior to the investigator's arrival, would first contact law enforcement to both request their scene photos and to ask about the first responders' findings. Additionally, the death investigator would request the Fire Rescue or Emergency Medical Services runsheet report in order to gather the missing data.

When a death call is received, the decision of whether "to go" or "not to go" to a scene may be determined by the investigator on duty, by the investigative supervisor, by the medical examiner/coroner on call, or by office policy and procedure. Some offices may require a scene visit for every violent death; others will visit the scene only by request of law enforcement. A good rule of thumb is to visit: (1) every scene suspicious for homicidal violence; (2) every infant death; (3) *all* decomposed remains; (4) at any request by law enforcement; and (5) on *any* additional case that cannot be explained by law enforcement to your satisfaction.

Death calls from a healthcare facility

The same information as listed previously must be collected because, depending on the nature of the case, any or all of these data could be important for triaging jurisdiction. The next question to be asked, after collecting all of the patient demographic data and that of the reporting entity, is "How did the decedent die?" The hospital *should* have an answer for this question such as "We think it is due to X ..." If X is natural, then the case will likely not reach jurisdictional criteria. If X is traumatic, toxicologic, or sudden/unexpected, the case will likely reach jurisdictional criteria. Cases in which the cause of death is natural (i.e., no evidence of acute/remote trauma or intoxication with a documented history of lethal natural disease) should immediately be elucidated so as to avoid wasting time of the hospital staff and the medical examiner/coroner staff. In some cases the hospital is calling to report the death because it is their policy, in other cases the attending physician wishes the case to be "run by the ME's office." Either is completely acceptable as it permits the medical examiner/coroner's office to examine these cases for occult jurisdictional criteria. If the case does not have a natural cause of death (i.e., sudden/unexpected death, trauma, or potentially intoxication related), when reporting the death, hospital staff should be aware of the course of patient care and should have the chart in their possession or have it be electronically accessible. If they are not familiar with the case or if they do not have access to the clinical data, it is appropriate to ask them to call back when they are familiar and after they have access to the clinical data. Reporting death is not something that is done quickly or something to be attempted with no preparation. As such, if the case is going to be properly triaged by medical examiner/coroner's staff, the reporting entity must be prepared to answer a series of probing questions. Answers from reporting entities, such as "I think ...," "I assume ...," or "I don't have that ...," are *unacceptable*. The data that are known by the hospital must be able to be conveyed to medical examiner/coroner's staff, otherwise the case cannot be triaged appropriately. In fact, the more prepared the reporting entity, the faster the triage will go. If the interpretation of the reporting hospital staff is suspect, confusing, or incomplete, it is also completely appropriate to ask to speak to the attending physician of the decedent, as they will be very familiar with the clinical course. If no one is available at that time who has knowledge of the clinical course of the decedent, again, it is completely appropriate to ask them to call back when they have the required information.

Most cases that reach jurisdictional criteria are clear

"The baby/child was found unresponsive at home and was pronounced dead within minutes of arrival to the emergency department" – clearly sudden and unexpected.

"The baby/child has injuries" – clearly violent.

"The baby/child has been in the hospital since birth due to maternal injuries and related obstetric complications suffered in a motor vehicle crash while still in utero" – clearly related to remote accidental maternal trauma.

Some of the cases will not be so clear

"The baby/child has been in the hospital since birth due to birth-related injuries." This has to be thoroughly questioned with regard to the use of the term "injuries." Conventionally, anoxia/hypoxia during the birthing process resulting in anoxic encephalopathy is considered a "birth injury" by medical personnel; however, parturition (childbirth), is not a benign process and sometimes it causes sublethal or lethal maternal or fetal stresses resulting in subsequent morbidity and mortality. Because childbirth is a *natural* process, any complication resulting from this *natural* process should be considered natural and should not reach jurisdictional criteria (depending on the jurisdictional governing rules). Alternatively, if the birth-related "injuries" are a consequence of maternal trauma or intoxication (i.e., pregnant mother sustained blunt force, sharp force, or gunshot-related injuries *or* was found to be positive for cocaine or methamphetamine [two drugs well known to cause placental complications and pre-term labor]), then the infant's postpartum complications and death (if considered to be related to the *in utero* insult), should be considered to reach jurisdictional criteria and the case should be brought in.

"The baby/child was neglected." This is a *very* open-ended opinion in the world of death certification as definitions of neglect are protean and myriad, usually based on one's own mores, morals, upbringing, and experience. The world of child protective services has its own definitions of "neglect" based on its own criteria that often have nothing to do with death certification. These cases can be difficult to triage effectively and unless it is an office policy to accept jurisdiction on these cases pro forma, a philosophical conundrum usually ensues. For the death investigator triaging this kind of case, it is always prudent to involve the forensic pathologist or coroner on call in order to permit them to ask questions and to assess the situation themselves. In this writer's experience, child protective services often will announce that they are investigating certain cases and will want the death investigation system to accept jurisdiction based on the preliminary assertion of neglect, rather than on an investigation based on objective facts. If child protective services and law enforcement are separate entities, law enforcement often relinquishes control of these investigations to child protective services, because it is commonly believed that child protective services are better able, and are better trained, to handle these kinds of investigations… However, this is completely dependent on the child protective services agency in question and should *not* be assumed out of hand. The reality is that protective services (whether adult or child) may be lackluster investigators and may not assist the death investigation system in investigating these cases at all. In addition, child protective services may hold their findings until the death investigation system finishes their investigation, which is counterproductive as the death investigation system requires investigatory information from all agencies involved to form their opinion(s). Thus cases of neglect have to be investigated knowing that there may be little to no ancillary assistance and, as such, as much preliminary information will have to be collected as early as possible in order to make a jurisdictional decision on the case and also to understand the parameters of the case and why neglect is being considered as a factor. The hospital that is reporting the case should be able to answer many, if not all, of your questions. If the reporting hospital cannot satisfactorily answer triage questions, the hospital should be able to direct the death investigator to the agency(ies) who are in charge of that arm of the investigation. There is no rush on the decision making and it may take a few hours to successfully navigate the personnel and circumstances, but the key is to take the burden of investigation on and figure out for yourself whether the case reaches your jurisdictional threshold rather than being told that it does by agencies that do not understand the parameters under which you work. Also, the investigative agencies may be under the misapprehension that an autopsy is going to answer all their investigatory questions, rather than actually collecting relevant circumstantial information for themselves.

"We think the death may be natural, but the parents (or caregivers) are being very evasive… or are giving us different stories." Following this statement, the next question asked by the death investigator should be "Have you informed the police?" If the hospital has informed the police, a detective should have been involved and their name and jurisdiction should be known to the hospital. The death investigator should contact the detective and interview them for relevant case information. If law enforcement has not been informed, the death investigator should instruct them to inform the police and have law enforcement begin their investigation. As in the case where a civilian calls in a death, the death investigator should make contact with the law enforcement agency responsible for investigating the death and inform them of what is known about the case and that you have instructed the hospital to make contact with them. At that point, law enforcement will likely make contact with the hospital and initiate an investigation on their own. In this way, the death investigation system becomes a nexus for the case to make sure that: (1) all the appropriate authorities are involved; and (2) that all involved are reporting their findings to the death investigation agency, which makes them far better informed about the case and the evolution of case information.

Documentation required from the reporting hospital

For many, if not all, infant or child cases being reported from the hospital, the information to request includes, but is not limited to, the following:

1. EMS runsheet (if available). Depending on the city/county, they may be available immediately to the hospital or the medical examiner/coroner's office or they may take time to be synthesized before they are deliverable. The medical examiner/coroner's office should have experience in requesting this information. Sometimes this information is crucial to the case and, as such, it should always be looked at as a potential treasure trove of investigatory data that can easily be overlooked.

2. Admission history and physical examination

   a. history of present illness
   b. past medical history, past surgical history, allergies, medications

c. exam findings/laboratories/imaging studies

d. assessment and plan.

3. Laboratory data

   a. basic metabolic panel
   b. complete blood count(s)
   c. toxicology screen(s)
   d. culture data.

4. Imaging studies

   – X-ray studies, CT scans, MRI scans, etc.

5. Reports of surgical procedures

   a. blood loss
   b. pre-/postoperative diagnoses
   c. injuries found
   d. evidence collected (i.e., bullets, bullet jackets, other foreign bodies, etc.).

6. Summary of hospital course

   a. in lieu of a discharge summary (as these are generally not prepared at the time of death)
   b. can be short, but should be complete and contain relevant information.

7. Expiration diagnosis(es)

   – Why did the person die?

For this information, when the hospital reporter is asked the cause of death, cardiac/respiratory arrest is *not* the answer. The question is the nature of the underlying disease, injury, or poison/intoxication that created the anatomic or physiologic injury culminating in death. If the hospital reporter does not know, then they should have access to the treating physician or their proxy to answer this question. In some cases, the cause of death is well characterized and, if natural and not related in any way to unnatural means (i.e., violence or drugs), will likely not meet jurisdictional criteria. If the answer is "we don't know," the treating physician should still be contacted to verify the clinical course and the jurisdictional decision can be made based on that information.

8. Death note

   – Information and/or time course of events leading to death. In some hospital systems, a death note must be written by the physician attending the death. In other systems it can be written by any staff member present to include nursing staff, religious clerics, or medical students.

9. Any police involvement (if known) and jurisdiction.

10. Admission blood (*whichever came first* and *before fluid resuscitation or transfusion of blood products*)

    – Remember, once fluids are started or blood products are transfused all plasma drug levels are decreased by dilution. In addition, plasma drug levels decrease due to metabolism over time, so the initial blood drawn is the very best sample for testing for toxicants in cases where time has elapsed from admission to death.

11. Attending physician's contact information for referral

    – Cell phone or pager number. This is usually listed under the physician's name on any of their progress notes. In addition, the nursing staff should always have a contact number for the treating physician(s), so the answer "I cannot contact him/her" is not satisfactory.

The death scene

Scene visitation

The components of any medicolegal death include a thorough "history" from the reporting entity, analysis of the death scene itself, the external examination of the dead body, the internal examination of the dead body, laboratory studies (i.e., bacterial or viral cultures, toxicology, metabolic panels, vitreous chemistry, etc.), and any investigative data generated through time by outside agencies (i.e., law enforcement, fire marshall, fire rescue, child or adult protective services, etc.).

As previously stated, the reporting entity is commonly law enforcement or a hospital and, as discussed earlier, the first report of death should include the decedent's name, age, date of birth, race, past medical history (if known), and the circumstances known regarding the death. In the case of law enforcement, they should have some investigative information as they have been at the scene for some time, have secured it, interviewed witnesses, at least preliminarily (if any exist), and, in the case of suspicious circumstances, have likely photographed the scene and collected the trace evidence left on scene, not associated with the body. They should have some idea as to the suspicion of injuries (although sometimes they have not yet approached the body), the presence of illegal drugs and paraphernalia, whether the scene was secure (were the doors and windows closed and locked?), and whether it appears as though there are any signs of "foul play" (valuables missing, drawers pulled out, or an appearance of the scene having been "rifled through" or "ransacked"). If possible, law enforcement should have visually identified the decedent, usually through comparison with the decedent's drivers license (if the face is exposed or if the body has been moved for resuscitative attempts). In addition, law enforcement should have taken an inventory of any medications that are present, which serves three functions: (1) it establishes a past medical history; (2) medication bottles contain an attending physician's name as a source to query

past medical history and as a source of medical record information; and (3) it can establish a potential cause of death either through the natural disease the medications were treating, or by the accidental or intentional overdose of the medication if the number of pills/capsules remaining appears to be fewer than there should be (or even completely absent). Inventory of the contents of the medication bottles may also imply a manner of death in cases where 30 tablets/capsules of medication were prescribed two days before with the direction to take one tablet per day, and only one or two pills remain. The findings in this example would imply the potential for an intentional overdose as one can mistakenly take one or two tablets, but not 20 or 30 at once. A caveat to using medication counts as a source of cause- or manner-specific information is that some people split medication up into smaller containers for daily reminder medication distribution or may even have sold some medication for profit. An additional caveat is that in some cases the decedent may have combined several prescriptions of the same medication type (e.g., one prescription of 15 oxycodone from one date and another prescription of 25 oxycodone from a different date – for a total of 40 oxycodone), so that the pill count is actually *more* than what they should have. In addition, with regard to medications, it is important to know what kind of medications are present in containers as some people may have combined prescriptions of different types of medications (e.g., 5 oxycodone, 3 hydrocodone, 10 GABApentin, and 17 atenolol); thus, in this example, there are more tablets/capsules than there likely should be in a bottle, but they are all different kinds and their raw numbers may or may not connote overdosage. Thus medication counts can be useful, but only in the context of all of the other case information provided.

The function of the medicolegal death investigator is *not* to recapitulate the police or firefighters' work product, but to focus on the dead body and how it came to be that way. Again, it is not the concern of the medicolegal death investigator *who* did it, rather their concern is whether the death was a result of actions of another person, actions by the victim themselves, unforeseen misfortune, or due to the decedent's own natural disease. Proper scene analysis, in fact, is the *primary resource* for the determination of cause and manner of death in most well-investigated cases. At the time the investigator leaves the scene, cause and manner should already be known to a reasonable degree of certainty and are only then confirmed by the pathologist during subsequent anatomic examination and laboratory analysis. There is far more to death scene investigation than standing about, taking photographs, and being in agreement that there is indeed a dead body present.

Death investigators have a central role to help define injury etiology, morphologic injury patterns, and association of putative weapon(s), if appropriate, so that police have some idea of what objects may be of evidentiary value *during the primary scene evaluation*. The information coming a day or days later, though still important, is potentially problematic as the specter of evidence contamination will be raised by defense experts later in court. The defense argument can be made that since the evidence was still "laying" at the potentially unsecured scene, and as such has been potentially accessible to "anyone" and potentially "contaminated" throughout that time, that the evidence should not be considered, despite any actual scientific value. This is a reasonable argument and is the exact reason why items of potential evidentiary value should be documented and secured as early as possible in death scene investigations.

Death investigators must also possess expertise in the assessment of postmortem changes not only in order to help determine postmortem interval but also to discriminate between injuries and normal decompositional changes.

Investigators must have good interpersonal skills as they interact with families of decedents, as well as police and fire rescue personnel, on a daily basis, and must know and respect their procedures and policies.

Investigators must also possess the medical skill set to allow them to communicate with healthcare officials using appropriate terminology to determine whether traumatic injuries, intoxicating agents, or natural disease have played a role in hospital-based deaths such that only appropriate cases are accepted and inappropriate cases are then released. They must be tenacious enough to ask probing questions, inquisitive enough to know what questions to ask, and well trained enough to recognize when their questions have been answered satisfactorily.

When the decision is made to go to the scene, the death scene investigators must first let law enforcement know that they are en route and that the body should not be touched any further. If the body is moved or taken out of the location, the scene has lost tremendous value, but is not completely useless at that point. It is usual and completely appropriate for first responders to assess unresponsive people for signs of life, as that is the primary and most important thing to do upon the discovery of an unresponsive human being. Upon assessment that the person is indeed dead (i.e., lack of pulse and respirations, cold to touch, palpable rigor mortis and/or developed livor mortis, skin sloughing, or decomposition/skeletonization), fire rescue should remove themselves from the scene and law enforcement should make their initial assessment as to the nature of the death. Depending on their training, experience, and their departmental policy and procedure, road patrol law enforcement officers (i.e., uniformed officers who are usually the first responders) may call homicide or major crimes detectives to come out, or road patrol may handle the case themselves. In either case, law enforcement should make their report of the death to the medical examiner/coroner's office as soon as possible in order to give investigators enough time to respond so as not to waste time. Additionally, it is appropriate and advisable for law enforcement to call the medical examiner/coroner's office to give them a courtesy "heads up" that they are en route to a death and that they will call back later with particulars. This will enable any death investigators involved (i.e., medicolegal death investigators, pathologists, medical examiners, or coroners) the ability to plan their day, evening, or early morning and to be able to decide whether they want to visit the scene *before* further alteration by law enforcement.

While still on the phone with law enforcement on scene, investigators should be assured of scene safety and security. Some scenes, depending on the circumstances, or the age or identity of the decedent, can be very explosive and may not be safe for unarmed personnel. In these cases, good sense and prudence must rule the day and provision must be made in office policy and procedure for the approved refusal to visit unsafe, unsecure scenes. The truth of the matter is that the decedent is dead and nothing is going to change the outcome at that point, so putting death investigators in danger just in order to photograph, diagram, and examine a dead body is inappropriate and ill advised. Police scene photographs can be used in place of death investigator photographs and the investigatory personnel get to stay safely away from potentially injurious or lethal situations.

Before leaving for the scene, the death investigator should assure that they possess personal protective equipment (i.e., sturdy non-porous gloves [latex or nitrile], Tyvek or other non-porous shoe covers or coveralls, safety goggles, and antibacterial cleanser for afterward) as well as documentation capability (i.e., camera with flash with data disk in place, thermometer, flash light, clipboard, writing instruments, scene diagram, and paper on which to make notes). The etiquette of investigators while on scene is based on personal preference, level of training and experience, and on office and law enforcement policies and procedures. In all cases, forensically prudent and mutually agreeable procedures must be utilized in order to examine and process these scenes appropriately.

On-scene behavior

Upon arrival at the scene death investigators should:

1. Park in an appropriate area, usually designated by law enforcement personnel.
2. Document the date and time of arrival.
3. Present identification at the crime scene tape or law enforcement checkpoint and make sure not only to make contact with the road patrol officer who is maintaining the scene log, but also to *ask for permission* to enter the scene (as defined by the crime scene tape).
4. Seek out and make contact with the lead detective or lead road patrol officer on scene.
5. Continue description of the circumstances of the case.
   (Adapted from Robinson and Trelka, 2011)

The discussion of circumstances should occur prior to, or during, entering the location so that the investigator is fully briefed on current information prior to entry to the death location. During the time it takes to drive to the scene location, information is constantly coming into the detectives and so the story may have significantly changed in that time frame. The circumstances should be completely reviewed and updated for clarity because the person who initially reported the

death may not have been fully informed or may have been mistaken. During this time the death investigator(s) can don their personal protective equipment and ready their camera and other materials in preparation for entering the death scene.

Photographic documentation can begin at this point by "putting the area on the map" using street signs or house numbers for subjects of photography. Law enforcement will have already photographed the scene, and those photos are usually available to the medical examiner/coroner's office if need be, so photography of minute external details is not necessary. Often detectives and crime scene personnel will follow death investigators in order to get a real-time description of what death investigators find and to permit photographs to be taken in an efficient manner. If there is anything that is noticed as compelling, the death investigator should ask if it was photographed by law enforcement. It may have been, or not. It gives law enforcement a chance to take another few photos of the item of interest, which may be integral to the case. The key of photography is to be able to place objects (including decedents) in space at the scene so that a clear narrative can be conveyed at a later date. Discussion with crime scene personnel can also help to determine if search criteria have to be adjusted. It is this author's experience that the body should not be approached quickly, rather photographs and thoughtful study and consideration of the surrounding environment may be crucial in interpreting the presence or absence of injuries and, if they exist, the injury type(s). It is important to remember that the body is not moving and that time, though important not to waste, is something that is available to you. There are systematic procedures that death investigators develop over time and experience that work for them. Procedures are mostly idiosyncratic and any elaborations on effective methods are certainly helpful, but "spiral circle" and "grid" methods are commonly used (Robinson and Trelka, 2011). Photo-documentation may include both taking pictures from points of reference in a 180-degree arc (Figure 5.1a through d) as well as documenting the location and position of the body using different angles and segmental approach photos (Robinson and Trelka, 2011).

In any event, approach photos up to the body to include several angles are an effective procedure. It should not have to be explained that it is inappropriate and ineffective to take close photographs with no orientation, or photographs from further away to give

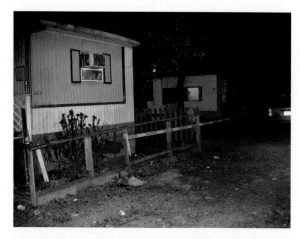

Figure 5.1a First of the 180-degree arc of photos of a death scene from outside the place of death.

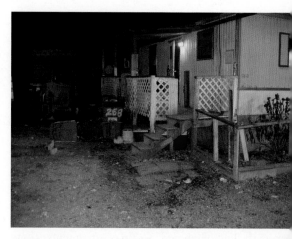

Figure 5.1b Second of the 180-degree arc of photos of a death scene from outside the place of death. The decedent's feet are visible in the left side of the photo.

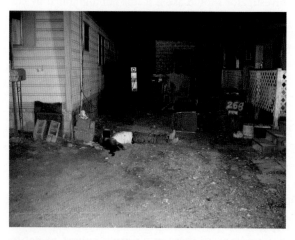

Figure 5.1c Third of the 180-degree arc of photos of a death scene from outside the place of death. The decedent is contained within the full frame of the photograph. Note the documentation of the area immediately surrounding the decedent.

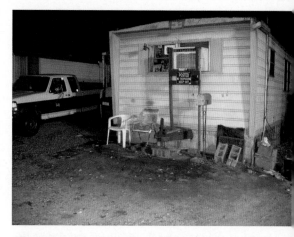

Figure 5.1d Fourth of the180-degree arc of photos of a death scene from outside the place of death. The decedent's head is visible in the bottom right of the photograph.

the close photographs context. Though you may have captured an important object or injury, if it cannot be traced in a photograph as to its spatial relationship to the scene and body, its importance is potentially lost.

Photographing the body should be done in a methodical way and usually begins with two or three orientation photos to capture the entire body in position. The goal is to eventually be able to have representative photos of all the body surfaces. A face photograph should also be taken (if the decedent is supine or near supine). If it is a homicide, photographs of the hands should be taken *before* any evidence is removed. If law enforcement has already taken hand photos and

done fingernail swabs/scrapings and gunshot residue lifts, taking further photos of the hands would only really be for documentation of injuries (i.e., scrimmage injuries from punching rough surfaces or incised and stab wounds consistent with "defensive injuries"). If a suicide, photographs of the hands, anterior wrists, and cubital fossae (i.e., inside elbows – a common place where blood is taken), should be captured to document the presence or absence of stigmata of previous suicide attempts. This simple act of documentation can help to direct the manner of death toward suicide if self-inflicted injuries, even those which may be sublethal, are present. In addition, when the body is manipulated, photographs should be taken of the body surfaces both clothed and with the clothing lifted away to expose the skin. *Prior to manipulation* of the body in any way, it is prudent to ask if you can touch the body, which gives crime scene personnel the option of reconsidering what they did, how they did it, and whether they wish to do anything additionally *before* the death investigator commits to touching the body. If the death investigator is permitted to examine the body, they may proceed in at least two ways, which are to: (1) continue taking their own photos while examining the body, which means potentially fouling the camera and/or the investigator's own face unless there are glove changes in between every photograph, and/or; (2) asking crime scene personnel to take photos either *for* the death investigator or *in lieu* of photography by the death investigator, after which the death investigator would get a copy of the crime scene photos the next day.

Examination of the body

The body, in the context of the death scene, is one of the most important items of evidence regarding the determination of cause and manner of death. The first thing that should be determined is whether the body is in the position where found, or whether the body had been moved in any way, shape, or form. If the body was moved (e.g., rolled over, "cut down," pulled away from the point of origin, examined for vital signs), the death investigator should find out who moved the body and speak to them immediately (if possible and in the presence of law enforcement) in order to determine the actual position of the body when found. In addition, it is important to establish whether any evidence had been collected from the body prior to the arrival and examination by the death investigator. If so, the death investigator should speak to the crime scene detective or forensic technician in order to determine what was found on the body (i.e., hairs/fibers, a knife, shell casings, a bullet, a ligature, a bag over the head, drugs or related paraphernalia, etc.).

The death investigator should also know *a priori* that the conditions in which the scene is contained may be poor due to weather, lighting, ambient temperature, or the watchful eyes of the public or the media and, as such, that all findings are to be considered *preliminary* until the body is examined and photographed in the well-illuminated confines of the autopsy suite.

When examining the body, all findings should be documented both in writing and photographically. In fact, were one wont to prioritize modalities of documentation, photography should come first and written record thereafter. The death investigator can always go back to the photos in order to clarify or further detail their findings after the examination is finished.

Documentation can be purely textual as in a narrative or bulleted list, or it can take the form of a diagram with illustrative props (i.e., furniture, appliances, walls, adjoining rooms, or other structures) indicated in spatial relationship to the body.

If the body is in a precarious position, it should be documented and then moved to an area where examination is possible with no danger of injury to live people or artifactual injury to the body from it slipping, falling, being incised, or being abraded by nearby objects. If the body must be moved, the area to which the body will be moved should be draped with a clean white sheet so that any trace evidence will not be lost in transport or during examination.

Following written and photo documentation of the general setting of the scene, the following steps should be taken:

1. Document the location of the body and description of how the body is positioned upon examination and, if different, how the body was found.
2. Document both the environment in which the body was found as well as its current environment (e.g., if the body was found floating in a canal, pool, or bathtub and was subsequently brought to shore).
3. Document the ambient conditions with temperature (always) and precipitation (if scene is outdoors).
4. Document the general features of the body (i.e., apparent race, sex, state of dress, and age).
5. Document the clothing (if any), type of clothing, and appropriateness of clothing (i.e., transgendered clothing, missing items from a usual location, added items in an unusual location, whether they are situated in the correct orientation, and any defects that may correspond or explain findings ascertained later in the physical examination).
6. Document the presence/absence of livor mortis (postmortem blood settling), on what surface it is apparent (i.e., anterior or posterior), and, upon

palpation, with photography, whether or not it blanches.

7. Document the presence/absence of rigor mortis (postmortem muscle stiffness) in the mandible, neck, trunk, and extremities with care to record in what limb(s) or structure(s) it exists and where it does not.

8. Document the hands by photography, with care, to visualize the entire dorsal and palmar surfaces in order to look for fingernail damage or "scrimmage"-type injuries, both of which may indicate that the decedent may have been in a physical struggle. The hand examination will permit the assessment of the hands for sharp-force injuries consistent with defensive-type injuries. In addition, the investigator should examine the wrists for acute injuries or healed scars consistent with acute suicidality or a remote suicidal attempt, respectively. If the law enforcement agency continues to practice the questionably forensically useful collection of gunshot residue (GSR), the hands can be sampled at this time as well. If the circumstances warrant it, fingernail swabs/cuttings can be procured at this time and receipted directly to law enforcement. If the circumstances warrant it, and law enforcement cannot or will not accept any evidence collection from the hands on scene, the hands can be covered with *paper* bags affixed externally to the wrist by rubber bands to protect any evidence from loss during transport.

9. Begin to palpate and examine the body for signs of injury or natural disease while also playing close attention to any evidentiary items that may be present. It is best to do this the same way every time in order to assure that nothing is overlooked. In whatever position the body is in, it is most logical to begin at the top of the head (cephalad) and move toward the feet (caudad). Note anything associated with the body (e.g., ligatures, bindings, weapons) and, if the decedent is clothed, be sure to *feel* the outside of all pockets *before* inserting a gloved hand into the pocket to determine if there is anything of interest in the pocket (i.e., identification, drugs or drug paraphernalia, a suicide note, particles of debris, etc.). Be sure to begin your examination in whatever position the body exists and, when

and if appropriate, turn the body over onto a clean white sheet for completion of the examination.

10. Document the conjunctivae, sclerae, and buccal (inside of the cheek and lip) mucosae for the presence of petechiae. Note that these are non-specific signs of venous congestion of the head and can occur passively (i.e., due to body position) or actively (i.e., due to thoracic or cervical compression during the antemortem or perimortem period, or even from elevated thoracic pressure exerted by the decedent before or during the dying process). Petechiae, if found, should be correlated with the scene; with further examination of the neck, thorax, and abdomen; any historical information from witnesses; the position of the body; and with first responders who may have attempted resuscitative efforts.

11. Examine the body underneath any items of clothing (i.e., lift up the shirt/blouse to examine the front and back of the trunk; visualize the abdomen; gently pull clothing away to uncover as much of the pelvis and buttocks as possible; examine the legs under shorts, slacks, or a skirt/dress; examine the feet including the soles of the feet and between the toes, etc.). Document any injuries, signs of natural disease, or that all is apparently unremarkable at that time with the knowledge that any ascertainment can and may be changed following closer examination in the autopsy suite. It may be forensically prudent, depending on the case, to remove some or all items of clothing as evidence for receipt to law enforcement at that time. This is a combination of personal preference, office and law enforcement policy, and using good forensic judgment and should *always* be considered as an option. The evidentiary utility of clothing that has been fouled by the passive leakage of blood, gastric contents, or fecal material, can approach zero, so careful thought should be given to removal of clothing and other evidence prior to transport of the body to avoid loss of, or obscuring, material evidence through transport of a clothed body. In cases of suspected criminal violence, if there are any compelling injuries or indicia of close contact with another person (i.e., suspect(s)), it is forensically prudent to

photo-document the area of interest with a scale (i.e., "L" shaped ruler authorized by the American Board of Forensic Odontology [ABFO]) and to collect evidence from the area with a sterile cotton-tipped swab followed by careful packaging and receipt to law enforcement.

12. Following examination and photo-documentation of all covered and uncovered surfaces, the body can be wrapped in a clean white sheet prior to insertion into a bodybag in order to physically separate the decedent from the bodybag itself and to contain any evidence that may still be adherent to, or associated with, the body.

13. Once the body has been placed in the bodybag, it is prudent, at least in all cases of suspected criminal violence or in cases of suspicious circumstance, to seal the bodybag with either a numbered plastic locking mechanism or at the very least with evidence tape that has been signed by the sealer. In either case, the seal should be photographed once complete in order to document that proper chain of custody is maintained.

14. Care should be given to gentle, controlled movement of the body in order to avoid any accidental postmortem traumatic artifacts (i.e., abrasions, lacerations, or "contusions," which may occur during vigorous transport, if the body is struck upon an inanimate object during transport, or if the body is inadvertently dropped due to weight, transport staff fatigue, or due to difficult extrication).

15. Following the completion of the examination and proper body disposition in a sealed bodybag, the death investigator should make contact with the lead detective prior to exiting the scene in order to both report any pertinent findings (i.e., with the caveat that opinions are subject to change upon further examination in the autopsy suite) and to ascertain whether any information has changed or has been updated since arrival. Thereafter, upon exit from the scene, the death investigator should make sure to inform the road patrol officer who is maintaining the scene log that you are leaving so they can reflect that in the record.

(Adapted from Clark *et al.*, 1996)

Infant death scene reconstruction

Death scenes for infants are somewhat specialized due to their relative anatomic and physiologic fragility. All of the elements previously discussed should be completed including the physical examination of the infant. Complete investigation of infant deaths entails a scene doll reconstruction (if permissible) utilizing a data collection survey or question battery. The investigative form from the Centers for Disease Control and Prevention (www.cdc.gov/sids/pdf/suidi-reporting-form.pdf) and Figure 5.2, or a similar question battery, should be utilized to direct the questions asked of the caregivers.

In addition, the actual surface on which the infant was found dead (i.e., couch, bed, crib, floor, mattress, car seat, etc.) with the actual bedding, blankets, pillows, etc., found positionally associated with the infant has to be visualized, photographed, and documented. As part of the reconstruction, an infant-sized doll should be used and then the death investigator will ask the witness(es) to demonstrate (using the doll) how the infant was positioned both when last known alive as well as when the infant was found dead (Figure 5.3a through g). The doll should be placed *exactly* as the witness(es) remember in the *same* positions (of last being known alive [Figure 5.3a] and when found dead [Figure 5.3b]) and using the *same* bedding and the *same* bedding-associated materials. Thus because of the requirement for the same associated materials and environment, the reconstruction should be completed (as permissible) as soon as is possible. Law enforcement presence should be requested to document the reconstruction for themselves and personally visualize the physical demonstration of placement of the doll representing the decedent.

Request of the scene doll reconstruction takes some thoughtful planning, and a tremendous amount of humility, as the death investigator is requesting the witness(es) to relive and reconstruct a tremendous stressor. The request should be made at an appropriate time with forethought and kindness. In addition, the request should be made with the *reasons* (in lay terms) why the reconstruction is being requested (i.e., that infants are generally unable to extricate themselves from potentially lethal positionally and mechanically challenging situations, as previously mentioned). This author has personally experienced many different emotional reactions (many unable to be predicted)

U.S. DEPARTMENT OF HEALTH AND HUMAN SERVICES
Centers for Disease Control and Prevention
Division of Reproductive Health
Maternal and Infant Health Branch
Atlanta, Georgia 30333

Sudden Unexplained Infant Death Investigation

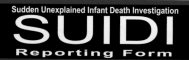

INVESTIGATION DATA

Infant's Last Name	Infant's First Name	Middle Name	Case Number

Sex: ___ Date of Birth: ___ Age: ___ SS#: ___

Race: [ ] White [ ] Black/African Am. [ ] Asian/Pacific Isl. [ ] Am. Indian/Alaskan Native [ ] Hispanic/Latino [ ] Other

Infant's Primary Residence:

Address: ___ City: ___ County: ___ State: ___ Zip: ___

Incident Address: ___ City: ___ County: ___ State: ___ Zip: ___

Contact Information for Witness:

Relationship to deceased: [ ] Birth Mother [ ] Birth Father [ ] Grandmother [ ] Grandfather

[ ] Adoptive or Foster Parent [ ] Physician [ ] Health Records [ ] Other Describe: ___

Last: ___ First: ___ M.: ___ SS#: ___

Address: ___ City: ___ State: ___ Zip: ___

Work Address: ___ City: ___ State: ___ Zip: ___

Home Phone: ___ Work Phone: ___ Date of Birth: ___

WITNESS INTERVIEW

1 Are you the usual caregiver?

[ ] No [ ] Yes

2 Tell me what happened:

3 Did you notice anything unusual or different about the infant in the last 24 hrs?

[ ] No [ ] Yes Specify: ___

4 Did the infant experience any falls or injury within the last 72 hrs?

[ ] No [ ] Yes Specify: ___

5 When was the infant LAST PLACED?

Date: ___ Military Time: ___ : ___ Location (room): ___

6 When was the infant LAST KNOWN ALIVE(LKA)?

Date: ___ Military Time: ___ : ___ Location (room): ___

7 When was the infant FOUND?

Date: ___ Military Time: ___ : ___ Location (room): ___

8 Explain how you knew the infant was still alive.

9 Where was the infant - (P)laced, (L)ast known alive, (F)ound (write **P**, **L**, or **F** in front of appropriate response)?

[ ] Bassinet	[ ] Bedside co-sleeper	[ ] Car seat	[ ] Chair
[ ] Cradle	[ ] Crib	[ ] Floor	[ ] In a person's arms
[ ] Mattress/box spring	[ ] Mattress on floor	[ ] Playpen	[ ] Portable crib
[ ] Sofa/couch	[ ] Stroller/carriage	[ ] Swing	[ ] Waterbed
[ ] Other - describe:			

Figure 5.2 The CDC SUIDI inventory (reproduced with permission from the CDC).

WITNESS INTERVIEW (cont.)

10 **In what position was the infant LAST PLACED?** ☐ Sitting ☐ On back ☐ On side ☐ On stomach ☐ Unknown
Was this the infant's usual position? ☐ Yes ☐ No What was the usual position? _____

11 **In what position was the infant LKA?** ☐ Sitting ☐ On back ☐ On side ☐ On stomach ☐ Unknown
Was this the infant's usual position? ☐ Yes ☐ No What was the usual position? _____

12 **In what position was the infant FOUND?** ☐ Sitting ☐ On back ☐ On side ☐ On stomach ☐ Unknown
Was this the infant's usual position? ☐ Yes ☐ No What was the usual position? _____

13 **Face position when LAST PLACED?** ☐ Face down on surface ☐ Face up ☐ Face right ☐ Face left

14 **Neck position when LAST PLACED?** ☐ Hyperextended (head back) ☐ Flexed (chin to chest) ☐ Neutral ☐ Turned

15 **Face position when LKA?** ☐ Face down on surface ☐ Face up ☐ Face right ☐ Face left

16 **Neck position when LKA?** ☐ Hyperextended (head back) ☐ Flexed (chin to chest) ☐ Neutral ☐ Turned

17 **Face position when FOUND?** ☐ Face down on surface ☐ Face up ☐ Face right ☐ Face left

18 **Neck position when FOUND?** ☐ Hyperextended (head back) ☐ Flexed (chin to chest) ☐ Neutral ☐ Turned

19 **What was the infant wearing?** *(ex. t-shirt, disposable diaper)* _____

20 **Was the infant tightly wrapped or swaddled?** ☐ No ☐ Yes - describe: _____

21 **Please indicate the types and numbers of layers of bedding both over and under infant (not including wrapping blanket):**

Bedding UNDER Infant	None	Number	Bedding OVER Infant	None	Number
Receiving blankets			Receiving blankets		
Infant/child blankets			Infant/child blankets		
Infant/child comforters (thick)			Infant/child comforters (thick)		
Adult comforters/duvets			Adult comforters/duvets		
Adult blankets			Adult blankets		
Sheets			Sheets		
Sheepskin			Pillows		
Pillows			Other, specify:		
Rubber or plastic sheet					
Other, specify:					

22 **Which of the following devices were operating in the infant's room?**
☐ None ☐ Apnea monitor ☐ Humidifier ☐ Vaporizer ☐ Air purifier ☐ Other - _____

23 **In was the temperature in the infant's room?** ☐ Hot ☐ Cold ☐ Normal ☐ Other - _____

24 **Which of the following items were near the infant's face, nose, or mouth?**
☐ Bumper pads ☐ Infant pillows ☐ Positional supports ☐ Stuffed animals ☐ Toys ☐ Other - _____

25 **Which of the following items were within the infant's reach?**
☐ Blankets ☐ Toys ☐ Pillows ☐ Pacifier ☐ Nothing ☐ Other - _____

26 **Was anyone sleeping with the infant?** ☐ No ☐ Yes

Name of individual sleeping with infant	Age	Height	Weight	Location in relation to infant	Imparement (intoxication, tired)

27 **Was there evidence of wedging?** ☐ No ☐ Yes - Describe: _____

28 **When the infant was found, was s/he:** ☐ Breathing ☐ Not Breathing
If not breathing, did you witness the infant stop breathing? ☐ No ☐ Yes

Figure 5.2 *(cont.)*

WITNESS INTERVIEW (cont.)

29 What had led you to check on the infant?

30 Describe the infant's appearance when found.

Appearance	Unknown	No	Yes	Describe and specify location
a) Discoloration around face/nose/mouth				
b) Secretions (foam, froth)				
c) Skin discoloration (livor mortis)				
d) Pressure marks (pale areas, blanching)				
e) Rash or petechiae (small, red blood spots on skin, membranes, or eyes)				
f) Marks on body (scratches or bruises)				
g) Other				

31 What did the infant feel like when found? *(Check all that apply.)*

☐ Sweaty ☐ Warm to touch ☐ Cool to touch ☐ Limp, flexible ☐ Rigid, stif ☐ Unknown

☐ Other - specify:

32 Did anyone else other than EMS try to resuscitate the infant? ☐ No ☐ Yes

Who? Date: Military time: :

33 Please describe what was done as part of resuscitation:

34 Has the parent/caregiver ever had a child die suddenly and unexpectedly? ☐ No ☐ Yes

Explain:

INFANT MEDICAL HISTORY

1 Source of medical information: ☐ Doctor ☐ Other healthcare provider ☐ Medical record ☐ Family

☐ Mother/primary caregiver ☐ Other:

2 In the 72 hours prior to death, did the infant have:

Condition	Unknown	No	Yes	Condition	Unknown	No	Yes
a) Fever				k) Apnea (stopped breathing)			
h) Diarrhea				e) Decrease in appetite			
b) Excessive sweating				l) Cyanosis (turned blue/gray)			
i) Stool changes				f) Vomiting			
c) Lethargy or sleeping more than usual				m) Seizures or convulsions			
j) Difficulty breathing				g) Choking			
d) Fussiness or excessive crying				n) Other, specify:			

3 In the 72 hours prior to death, was the infant injured or did s/he have any other condition(s) not mentioned?

☐ No ☐ Yes - describe:

4 In the 72 hours prior to the infants death, was the infant given any vaccinations or medications? ☐ No ☐ Yes

(Please include any home remedies, herbal medications, prescription medicines, over-the-counter medications.)

Name of vaccination or medication	Dose last given	Date given Month	Day	Year	Approx. time (Military Time)	comments:
1.						
2.						
3.						
4.						

Figure 5.2 *(cont.)*

INFANT MEDICAL HISTORY (cont.)

5 **At any time in the infant's life, did s/he have a history of?**

Medical history	Unknown	No	Yes	Describe
a) Allergies *(food, medication, or other)*				
b) Abnormal growth or weight gain/loss				
c) Apnea *(stopped breathing)*				
d) Cyanosis *(turned blue/gray)*				
e) Seizures or convulsions				
f) Cardiac *(heart)* abnormalities				

6 **Did the infant have any birth defects(s)?** ☐ No ☐ Yes

Describe:

7 **Describe the two most recent times that the infant was seen by a physician or health care provider:**
(Include emergency department visits, clinic visits, hospital admissions, observational stays, and telephone calls)

	First most recent visit	Second most recent visit
a) Date		
b) Reason for visit		
c) Action taken		
d) Physician's name		
e) Hospital/clinic		
f) Address		
g) City		
h) State, ZIP		
i) Phone number		

8 **Birth hospital name:** _____ Discharge date: _____

Street address: _____

City: _____ State: _____ Zip: _____

9 **What was the infant's length at birth?** _____ inches or _____ centimeters

10 **What was the infant's weight at birth?** _____ pounds _____ ounces or _____ grams

11 **Compared to the delivery date, was the infant born on time, early, or late?**

☐ On time ☐ Early - how many weeks? _____ ☐ Late - how many weeks? _____

12 **Was the infant a singleton, twin, triplet, or higher gestation?**

☐ Singleton ☐ Twin ☐ Triplet ☐ Quadrupelet or higher gestation

13 **Were there any complications during delivery or at birth?** *(emergency c-section, child needed oxygen)* ☐ Yes ☐ No

Describe:

14 **Are there any alerts to the pathologist?** *(previous infant deaths in family, newborn screen results)* ☐ Yes ☐ No

Specify:

Figure 5.2 *(cont.)*

INFANT DIETARY HISTORY

1 On what day and at what approximate time was the infant last fed?

Date: [____] Military Time: [____]:[____]

2 What is the name of the person who last fed the infant? [____]

3 What is his/her relationship to the infant? [____]

4 What foods and liquids was the infant fed in the <u>last 24 hours</u> (include last fed)?

Food	Unknown	No	Yes	Quantity (ounces)	Specify: (type and brand)
a) Breast milk (one/both sides, length of time)					
b) Formula (brand, water source - ex. Similac, tap water)					
c) Cow's milk					
d) Water (brand, bottled, tap, well)					
e) Other liquids (teas, juices)					
f) Solids					
g) Other					

5 Was a new food introduced in the 24 hours prior to his/her death? [ ] No [ ] Yes
If yes, describe (ex. content, amount, change in formula, introduction of solids)

[____]

6 Was the infant last placed to sleep with a bottle? [ ] Yes [ ] No - if no, skip to question **9** below

7 Was the bottle propped? (i.e., object used to hold bottle while infant feeds) [ ] No [ ] Yes

If yes, what object was used to prop the bottle? [____]

8 What was the quantity of liquid (in ounces) in the bottle? [____]

9 Did the death occur during? [ ] Breast-feeding [ ] Bottle-feeding [ ] Eating solid foods [ ] Not during feeding

10 Are there any factors, circumstances, or environmental concerns that may have impacted the infant that have not yet been identified? (ex. exposed to cigarette smoke or fumes at someone else's home, infant unusually heavy, placed with positional supports or wedges)

[ ] No [ ] Yes

If yes, - describe: [____]

PREGNANCY HISTORY

1 Information about the infant's birth mother:

First name: [____] Last name: [____]
Middle name: [____] Maiden name: [____]
Birth date: [____] SS#: [____]

Street address: [____] City: [____] State: [____] Zip: [____]

How long has the birth mother been at this address? Years: [____] Months: [____]

Previous Address: [____]

2 At how many weeks or months did the birth mother begin prenatal care? [ ] No parental care [ ] Unknown

Weeks: [____] Months: [____]

3 Where did the birth mother receive prenatal care? (Please specify physician or other health care provider name and address.)

Physician/provider: [____] Hospital/clinic: [____] Phone: [____]

Street address: [____] City: [____] State: [____] Zip: [____]

Figure 5.2 (cont.)

PREGNANCY HISTORY (cont.)

4 At how many weeks or months did the birth mother begin prenatal care? ☐ No ☐ Yes
(ex. high blood pressure, bleeding, gestational diabetes)

Specify: _____

5 Was the birth mother injured during her pregnancy with the infant? *(ex. auto accident, falls)* ☐ No ☐ Yes

Specify: _____

6 During her pregnancy, did she use any of the following?

	Unknown	No	Yes	Daily		Unknown	No	Yes	Daily
a) Over the counter medications					d) Cigarettes				
b) Prescription medications					e) Alcohol				
c) Herbal remedies					f) Other				

7 Currently, does any caregiver use any of the following?

	Unknown	No	Yes	Daily		Unknown	No	Yes	Daily
a) Over the counter medications					d) Cigarettes				
b) Prescription medications					e) Alcohol				
c) Herbal remedies					f) Other				

INCIDENT SCENE INVESTIGATION

1 Where did the incident or death occur? _____

2 Was this the primary residence? ☐ No ☐ Yes

3 Is the site of the incident or death scene a daycare or other childcare setting? ☐ Yes ☐ No - If no, skip to question **8**

4 How many children (under age 18) were under the care of the provider at the time of the incident or death? _____

5 How many adults (age 18 and over) were supervising the child(ren)? _____

6 What is the license number and licensing agency for the daycare?

License number: _____ Agency: _____

7 How long has the daycare been open for business? _____

8 How many people live at the site of the incident or death scene?

Number of adults (18 years or older): _____ Number of children (under 18 years old): _____

9 Which of the following heating or cooling sources were being used? *(Check all that apply)*

☐ Central air	☐ Gas furnace or boiler	☐ Wood burning fireplace	☐ Open window(s)
☐ A/C window unit	☐ Electric furnace or boiler	☐ Coal burning furnace	☐ Wood burning stove
☐ Ceiling fan	☐ Electric space heater	☐ Kerosene space heater	☐ Floor/table fan
☐ Electric baseboard heat	☐ Electric (radiant) ceiling heat	☐ Window fan	☐ Unknown

☐ Other - specify: _____

10 Indicate the temperature of the room where the infant was found unresponsive:

☐ Thermostat setting ☐ Thermostat reading ☐ Actual room temp. ☐ Outside temp.

11 What was the source of drinking water at the site of the incident or death scene? *(Check all that apply.)*

☐ Public/municipal water ☐ Bottled water ☐ Well ☐ Unknown ☐ Other - Specify: _____

12 The site of the incident or death scene has: *(check all that apply)*

☐ Insects	☐ Mold growth	☐ Smoky smell *(like cigarettes)*
☐ Pets	☐ Dampness	☐ Presence of alcohol containers
☐ Peeling paint	☐ Visible standing water	☐ Presence of drug paraphenalia
☐ Rodents or vermin	☐ Odors or fumes - Describe:	_____

☐ Other - specify: _____

13 Describe the general appearance of incident scene: *(ex. cleanliness, hazards, overcrowding, etc.)*

Specify: _____

Figure 5.2 *(cont.)*

INVESTIGATION SUMMARY

1 Are there any factors, circumstances, or environmental concerns about the incident scene investigation that may have impacted the infant that have not yet been identified?

2 Arrival times

Military time

Law enforcement at scene: :

DSI at scene: :

Infant at hospital: :

Investigator's Notes

1 Indicate the task(s) performed

☐ Additional scene(s)? (forms attached)

☐ Doll reenactment/scene re-creation

☐ Photos or video taken and noted

☐ Materials collected/evidence logged

☐ Referral for counseling

☐ EMS run sheet/report

☐ Notify next of kin or verify notification

☐ 911 tape

2 If more than one person was interviewed, does the information differ? ☐ No ☐ Yes

If yes, detail any differences, inconsistencies of relevant information: *(ex. placed on sofa, last known alive on chair.)*

INVESTIGATION DIAGRAMS

1 Scene Diagram:

2 Body Diagram:

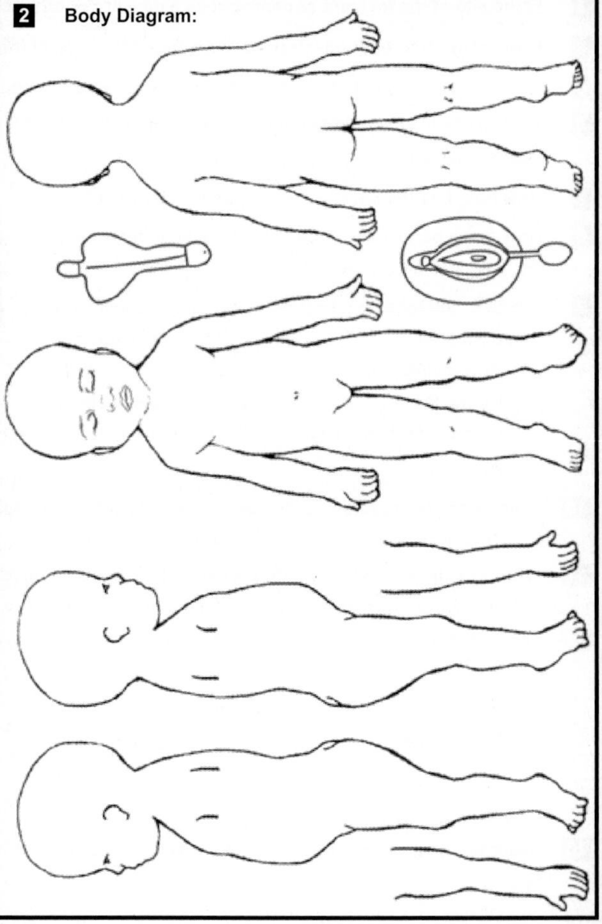

Page 7

Figure 5.2 *(cont.)*

SUMMARY FOR PATHOLOGIST

Case Information

1 **Investigator information** Name: [ ] Agency: [ ] Phone: [ ]

Date | Military time
Investigated: [ ] :
Pronounced dead: [ ] :

2 **Infant's information:** Last: [ ] First: [ ] M: [ ] Case #: [ ]

Sex: [ ] Male [ ] Female Date of Birth: [ ] Age: [ ]

Race: [ ] White [ ] Black/African Am. [ ] Asian/Pacific Islander

[ ] Am. Indian/Alaskan Native [ ] Hispanic/Latino [ ] Other: [ ]

Sleeping Environment

1 **Indicate whether preliminary investigation suggests any of the following:**

Yes No

[ ][ ] Asphyxia *(ex. overlying, wedging, choking, nose/mouth obstruction, re-breathing, neck compression, immersion in water)*
[ ][ ] Sharing of sleep surface with adults, children, or pets
[ ][ ] Change in sleep condition *(ex. unaccustomed stomach sleep position, location, or sleep surface)*
[ ][ ] Hyperthermia/Hypothermia *(ex. excessive wrapping, blankets, clothing, or hot or cold environments)*
[ ][ ] Environmental hazards *(ex. carbon monoxide, noxious gases, chemicals, drugs, devices)*
[ ][ ] Unsafe sleep condition *(ex. couch/sofa, waterbed, stuffed toys, pillows, soft bedding)*

Infant History

[ ][ ] Diet *(e.g., solids introduced, etc.)*
[ ][ ] Recent hospitalization
[ ][ ] Previous medical diagnosis
[ ][ ] History of acute life-threatening events *(ex. apnea, seizures, difficulty breathing)*
[ ][ ] History of medical care without diagnosis
[ ][ ] Recent fall or other injury
[ ][ ] History of religious, cultural, or ethnic remedies
[ ][ ] Cause of death due to natural causes other than SIDS *(ex. birth defects, complications of preterm birth)*

Family Info

[ ][ ] Prior sibling deaths
[ ][ ] Previous encounters with police or social service agencies
[ ][ ] Request for tissue or organ donation
[ ][ ] Objection to autopsy

Exam

[ ][ ] Pre-terminal resuscitative treatment
[ ][ ] Death due to trauma (injury), poisoning, or intoxication

Investigator Insight

[ ][ ] Suspicious circumstances
[ ][ ] Other alerts for pathologist's attention

Any "Yes" answers above should be explained in detail (description of circumstances):

Pathologist

2 **Pathologist information** Name: [ ]

Agency: [ ] Phone: [ ] Fax: [ ]

37

Figure 5.2 *(cont.)*

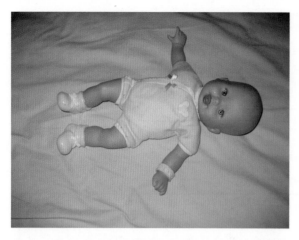

Figure 5.3a Re-enactment doll placed as "last seen alive" in crib.

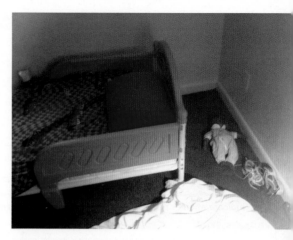

Figure 5.3b Re-enactment doll placed as "found" on floor in between bed and wall.

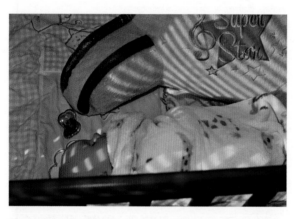

Figure 5.3c Photo from long edge of crib of re-enactment doll placed as "found."

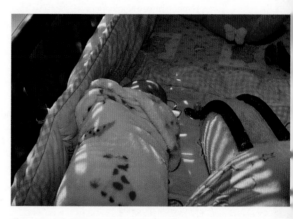

Figure 5.3d Photo from end of crib of re-enactment doll placed as "found".

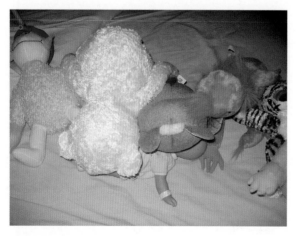

Figure 5.3e Re-enactment doll placed as "found" underneath toys arranged in the crib.

to the request, and cannot stress enough how sensitive the death investigator and law enforcement personnel must be in these situations.

The positions and all material around the infant must be photographed and documented (Figures 5.3c through e).

In addition, if the infant was co-sleeping with other children or adult caregivers, the doll must be placed (if permissible) with those involved on the sleep surface (i.e., sofa, bed, chair, etc.) in order to show the spatial relationships between the co-sleepers and the infant (Figure 5f and g).

The re-enactment should be carried out within reason and as permissible as these situations can be emotionally charged, and investigators must work within the confines of decency and avoid undue emotional

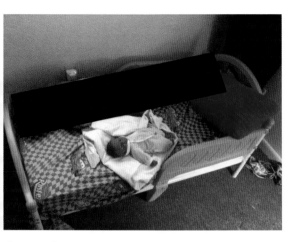

Figure 5.3f Re-enactment doll "laid to sleep" next to pre-adolescent co-sleeper.

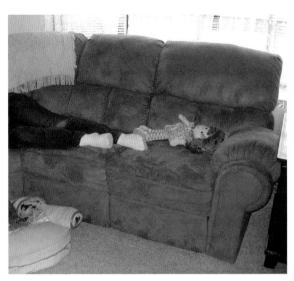

Figure 5.3g Re-enactment doll placed as "found" at adult caregivers feet on a sectional sofa.

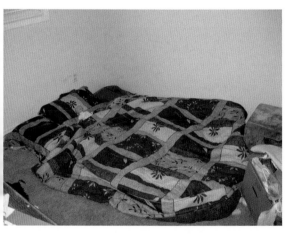

Figure 5.4a Re-enactment doll placed as "last seen alive" on adult air mattress with full-size bed clothes.

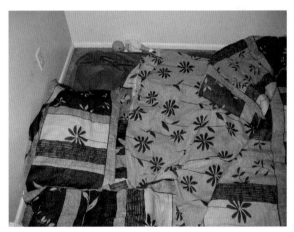

Figure 5.4b Re-enactment doll placed as "found" on the floor between the air mattress and the wall.

stress on family members or caregivers who have just lost a loved one. Special care must be taken to speak to the caregivers who last saw the infant alive, and recording all relevant circumstances, as well as to the person who found the infant dead or in terminal distress, as well as noting all the relevant circumstances. These can be even more emotionally charged than an adult death for obvious reasons.

The purpose of the doll reconstruction is to attempt to ascertain whether position, entrapment, or co-sleeping may have played a role in the death (Figure 5.4a through f). The pathologist, medical examiner, or coroner may be invited and, depending on office policy and procedure, their presence may be compulsory. For cases of child or adolescent death, scene visitation may be probative, but it will depend on the case and the circumstances.

Scene report writing

A scene report should contain all of the material demographic information collected in a case (as shown in Figure 5.5). These documents are generally discoverable, so the information collected and any opinions rendered should be completely factual (based on the information available at that time), defensible, and stated as preliminary.

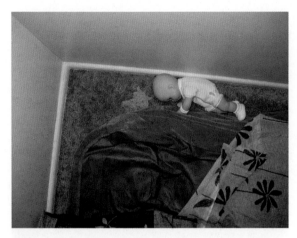

Figure 5.4c Closer photograph of re-enactment doll placed as "found" on the floor between the air mattress and the wall. Note the puddle of dried vomit on the carpet near the head of the doll. This corroborated the true position of the decedent.

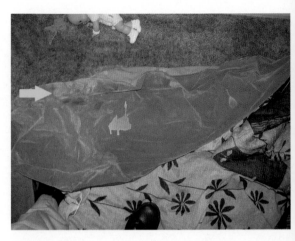

Figure 5.4d Re-enactment doll in place with edge of air mattress pulled back to expose the side that would have faced the decedent. Notice the patterned stain at the tip of the arrow.

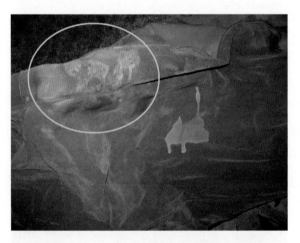

Figure 5.4e Closer photograph of patterned stain (circled) on edge of mattress. The color and texture are consistent with the vomit on the carpet and that found on the face and clothing of the actual decedent.

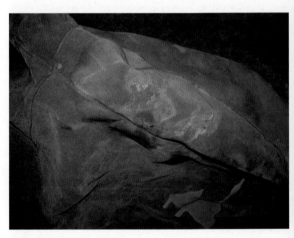

Figure 5.4f Close photograph of the patterned stain on the edge of the air mattress. The shape is most consistent with the decedent's facial features to include a closed eye (upper left), a nose with naris voids, and patterning under the nose consistent with the decedent's mouth.

Hospital visitation

In certain cases (e.g., death is upon arrival at the hospital), it may be important to visit the hospital to examine the decedent (especially in infant deaths) before transport to the medical examiner/coroner's office. In infant deaths, visiting the hospital permits death investigators to speak with law enforcement (who are usually present) and to interview parents/caregivers of the infant (who are usually also present) earlier, rather than waiting to try to contact them as they are traveling between the hospital, home, to church/temple, family member's houses, and/or funeral homes. In fact, it is often very difficult to make contact with the family of decedents of any age group after a certain amount of time has transpired after the death. There are so many issues that arise for them, so many duties to be performed, and so much emotional and spiritual support that is rendered, that attempting contact can be fruitless for hours or even days following the death. Therefore when speaking to the reporting agency (i.e., hospital or law enforcement), it is important that they are told that a death investigator will be en route to

XXXX COUNTY MEDICAL EXAMINER
Address
Phone number

SCENE INVESTIGATION

NAME: AUTOPSY NO:
- -

DATE OF SCENE:

ADDRESS:

INVESTIGATOR/PATHOLOGIST:

NOTIFICATION OF SCENE (WHO/DATE/TIME):

INITIAL DISCUSSION WITH POLICE (WHO/WHEN):

REASON FOR POLICE CONSULTATION:

TIME DISPATCHED TO SCENE FROM HOME/OFFICE:

ARRIVAL AT SCENE:

POINT(S) OF CONTACT:

VITAL STATISTICS OF DECEDENT:

LAST KNOWN ALIVE:

DISCOVERED DEAD:

PRONOUNCED DEAD:

CPR ATTEMPTED:

DEPARTURE FROM SCENE:

ARRIVAL AT HOME/OFFICE:

AUTOPSY SCHEDULED:

Figure 5.5 Scene visitation report template.

the hospital to examine the decedent, collect information, medical records (if any), and clinical data *prior* to decedent transport. This enables information transfer from medical personnel to the death investigator, and also gives the opportunity for law enforcement and the death investigation system to interview caregivers independently, but relatively contemporaneously.

Upon arrival at the hospital, the death investigator should make contact with the charge nurse or attending physician and with the lead detective attached to the case. The medical and law enforcement agencies should give their case information and enable the death investigator to ask any questions they have. Additional inquiries to the normal investigatory questions are: (1) the temperature of the decedent; and (2) the presence (if any) of rigor and livor mortis upon arrival. This can be very important information for correlation with the caregiver's information regarding the death and pre-hospital circumstances. The death investigator should then be shown to the decedent, at which time photo documentation of the decedent should take place and the decedent should be examined in the presence of law enforcement and the attending physician so that any questions about physical findings can be immediately answered and law enforcement has immediate feedback. There may be discussion of physical findings or imaging by the hospital staff, to which the death investigator should reply that *all findings will be evaluated at autopsy*. This is a safe reply to findings reported by medical personnel as hospital imaging modalities are fantastic tools, but are not as sensitive as autopsy for finding certain lesions, injuries, and physical signs, thus all findings reported by hospital staff will be evaluated, interpreted, and documented at autopsy.

The investigator should then interview the parent(s)/caregiver(s)/witness(es) present in order to document their information. This interview can be performed independent of law enforcement in order to check agreement with what the parent(s)/caregiver(s) told law enforcement in their interview. In addition, because the medical examiner/coroner's office is a medical office, has medical concerns, and does not have any power of criminal investigation or arrest, people may tell death investigators more sensitive information than they will offer to law enforcement. This is no value judgment on law enforcement, it is merely a fact that this author has found on numerous occasions wherein witnesses, parents, and caregivers will often disclose to death investigators more personal or sensitive information than they will to law enforcement personnel.

After the parent(s)/caregiver(s) are interviewed, in the case of infant death, the death investigator should begin collecting information via the aforementioned SUID inventory (or one like it) and should request the scene doll reconstruction. The death investigator should, as previously mentioned, explain the logic behind the reconstruction and that it should be performed as soon as possible. In this way the parent(s)/caregiver(s) have an opportunity to think about it, can ask questions directly to the death investigator, and the reconstruction can commence soon after leaving the hospital in order to assure that all of the relevant materials will be present unchanged, which may not be possible if significant time elapses from infant death to scene doll reconstruction.

In cases where there is suspicion of violence or criminal activity, the hospital visit also provides the death investigator with an opportunity to document any evidence still present on the infant before it is impounded by law enforcement. If there is any evidence, it should be collected by law enforcement rather than having it be transported via bodybag, or in a paper bag, from the hospital to the medical examiner/coroner's office only to be turned over to law enforcement later. Remember, the key to evidence handling is to keep the chain of custody as short as possible – so that as few people as possible have had possession, care, and control of the evidence.

Once finished at the hospital, the findings should be textually documented, but not in a scene report, since the scene has not yet been visited. If a reconstruction is going to occur, then following documentation of the reconstruction, all relevant information can be documented in a scene doll reconstruction report (which should take the form of the CDC SUID inventory with supportive photo documentation).

Post-scene evaluations

Introduction

The National Association of Medical Examiners (NAME) has written several guiding documents on the procedures and policies required from medicolegal death investigators, forensic pathologists, medical examiners, and coroners. NAME Forensic Autopsy Performance Standards (NAME, 2015) "Standard B3: Selecting Deaths Requiring Forensic Autopsies," states that officers responsible for medicolegal death investigation have been established to safeguard the public. NAME maintains that certain deaths (i.e., by criminal violence, of children, due to a device accessible to the public, or in police custody, etc.) can arouse public interest, raise questions, or engender mistrust of authority. In addition, NAME maintains that there are specific types of circumstances in which a forensic autopsy provides the best opportunity for competent investigation, including those decedents who require scientific identification, decomposed remains, those found in bodies of water, bodies burned beyond recognition, and people who have died from workplace injuries. Performance of autopsies in these cases protects the interests of the public and documents findings able to address legal, public health, and public safety concerns. For categories other than those listed below, the decision to perform an autopsy involves professional discretion or is dictated by local guidelines. For the categories excerpted from NAME Forensic Autopsy Performance Standards and listed below, NAME maintains that public interest is so compelling that one must always assume that questions can and will arise that require information obtainable *only* by forensic autopsy. The forensic pathologist shall perform a forensic autopsy when:

B3.1 the death is known or suspected to have been caused by apparent criminal violence.

B3.2 the death is unexpected and unexplained in an infant or child.

B3.3 the death is associated with police action.

B3.4 the death is apparently non-natural and in custody of a local, state, or federal institution.

B3.5 the death is due to acute workplace injury.

B3.6 the death is caused by apparent electrocution.

B3.7 the death is by apparent intoxication by alcohol, drugs, or poison, unless a significant interval has passed and the medical findings and absence of trauma are well documented.

B3.8 the death is caused by unwitnessed or suspected drowning.

B3.9 the body is unidentified and the autopsy may aid in identification.

B3.10 the body is skeletonized.

B3.11 the body is charred.

B3.12 the forensic pathologist deems a forensic autopsy is necessary to determine cause or manner of death, or document injuries/disease, or collect evidence.

B3.13 the deceased is involved in a motor vehicle incident and an autopsy is necessary to document injuries and/or determine the cause of death.

NAME Forensic Autopsy Standards are clear in stating that the:

(1) Forensic autopsy is considered the practice of medicine.

(2) Autopsies should be performed by a licensed forensic pathologist or a physician who is a forensic pathologist in-training (i.e., resident/fellow).

(3) The quality of the autopsy rests solely on the forensic pathologist who must *directly* supervise staff.

(4) Allowing non-forensic pathologists to conduct forensic autopsy procedures without *direct* supervision and guidance is fraught with the potential for serious errors and omission.

(5) Autopsy performance includes the discretion to determine the need for additional dissection techniques and laboratory testing.

NAME Forensic Autopsy Performance Standards direct:

(1) The forensic pathologist or residents in pathology perform all autopsies.
(2) The forensic pathologist *directly* supervises all assistance rendered during postmortem examinations.
(3) The forensic pathologist or residents in pathology perform all dissections of removed organs.
(4) The forensic pathologist determines need for special dissections or additional testing.
(5) The forensic pathologist *shall not perform* more than 325 autopsies in a year; the recommended maximum number is 250 per year.

Thus to be in agreement with NAME standards, offices must follow these directives, but, as appropriate, there is some clear latitude as required.

NAME also directs that:

(1) Interpretation and opinions related to death investigations are formulated after accumulation and review of all material information available at the time of the death investigation and that the forensic pathologist is in charge of all of these activities.
(2) The forensic pathologist reviews and interprets all data from laboratory assays requested and reviews all ancillary and consultative reports (as discussed in detail below).
(3) The determination of cause and manner of death should rest in the hands of the forensic pathologist (however, in coroner jurisdictions, the coroner is empowered to make those determinations).

External examination versus autopsy

There are reasons that external examination is appropriate over autopsy (as long as the aforementioned NAME criteria are not met). If the death is non-criminal and a cause is clear from the external examination (i.e., multiple blunt force injuries from an automobile crash, accidental penetrating injuries, injuries resulting from clear suicidal intent, etc.) *or* if the death is due to non-criminal trauma (e.g., near drown-

ing, multiple blunt force injuries) or natural diseases (e.g., anatomic aberrations, naturally acquired infections, or metabolic disorders well characterized in a medical record or clear by physical examination) and the decedent has had a well-characterized admission into a hospital and the medical records are made available for review to the forensic pathologist, external examination is completely appropriate and fiscally responsible.

When external examination is selected over autopsy, certain documentation should be assured for anticipated retrospective review, such as radiographs illustrative of the cause of death (as appropriate), photographs illustrative of the cause of death (as appropriate), and saved medical records that document the non-suspicious/non-criminal anatomic and/or physiologic aberration that culminated in, or is contributory to, death. If the cause of death is unclear in any way *or* if the decision of cause of death is reasonably between two potential causes, then an autopsy should logically be performed. The autopsy, in fact, should be the baseline means of determining cause and manner of death at the exclusion of clear and obvious non-criminal etiologies.

Law enforcement presence at examination

It is generally completely up to the forensic pathologist, medical examiner, or coroner as to the permissibility of law enforcement to be present during postmortem examination. Some offices have a very wide-open policy and permit not only detectives to be present during the examination of their appointed case(s), but also law enforcement trainees, attorneys, attorney trainees, medical students, and medical residents. There are some offices in which no extraneous personnel are permitted in the autopsy suite during examination, regardless of their relationship to the case. This is reasonable in light of the wont to reduce the aforementioned "specter of contamination." There are still other offices where, despite a rather open policy for law enforcement to be present for postmortem examinations, law enforcement declines to be present for various reasons.

This writer has found the presence of law enforcement personnel, especially the lead detective and forensic technicians/forensic detectives, to be a boon during postmortem examination in that a "real-time" updated circumstantial history can be given during the examination, findings can be related to law enforcement personnel with immediate real-time feedback, and law enforcement personnel are then able to ask questions and have answers in real-time. In addition, the presence of law enforcement personnel permits evidence transfer to occur directly from pathologist to the police agency so that the chain of custody is as short as possible. It appears to this writer that the case is tremendously benefitted and occasionally *outright solved* by the presence of law enforcement in the autopsy suite during postmortem examination and respectful, thoughtful resonance between the forensic pathologist and various police agencies.

Preliminary procedures

All *available* investigatory and medical information is reviewed prior to external examination and autopsy. All, some, or none of the pertinent information may be known or available at the time of autopsy and, as such, each case is going to come with various levels of historical information. Historical information directs and informs autopsy performance as to areas of interest and anticipates special procedures, preliminary information answers questions unique to the case, and enables the informed documentation of evidence that may have been overlooked, or packaged with the personal effects, had the pathologist not been made aware of its importance *a priori*. In total, the forensic pathologist should know and have reviewed all that is knowable and reviewable *prior* to the commencement of the external examination, in order to direct the procedures of the autopsy to answer the idiosyncratic questions of the case.

NAME Autopsy Standards direct that the forensic pathologist:

(1) Reviews the circumstances of death prior to forensic autopsy.
(2) Measures or causes to be measured and recorded the decedent's body length and body weight.
(3) Examines the external aspects of the body before internal examination.
(4) Photographs, or causes to be photographed, and describes the decedent as presented (i.e., "as is") to the office.
(5) Documents and correlates clothing findings with injuries of the body in criminal cases.

(6) Identifies and collects or causes to be collected trace evidence on clothing in criminal cases.
(7) Removes or causes to be removed the clothing.
(8) Photographs and lists or causes to be photographed and listed clothing and personal effects.

The forensic pathologist will document the apparent age of the decedent or will take and record measurements used in the establishment of the age of the decedent. The forensic pathologist will inspect and describe the sex, the racial characteristics, the hair, the eyes (i.e., irides, corneae, sclerae, and conjuctivae), any abnormalities in body habitus, scars, tattoos, skin exanthema, or congenital/acquired anatomic variations, the presence and quality or absence of dentition, the head, neck, thorax, abdomen, extremities, the genitals, and posterior body surfaces, and any evidence of medical or surgical interventions. In addition, the pathologist will inspect and describe the livor and rigor mortis, any postmortem changes, evidence of embalming, and any decompositional changes.

Special procedures and evidence collection

Radiography

Not all cases require radiography; however, new technology has come to the fore, which makes pre-examination radiography simple and temporally efficient. There are radiography machines capable of anterior/posterior full body radiographic survey in less than one minute. Lateral survey can be completed in a relative piecemeal fashion in the same time frame. Using this kind of technology, every decedent brought in can be surveyed for occult trauma, and occult natural disease states can be appreciated on a wider array of decedents. Radiographic survey can detect and localize penetrating injuries, projectiles, foreign objects, radio-opaque evidence of all types, and can help to document surgical devices that can assist in identification of remains that are otherwise unrecognizable (i.e., decomposed, post-anthropophagy, or burned beyond recognition). NAME directs that the forensic pathologist or their representative shall make or have made a radiographic survey of all infants, all explosion victims, all gunshot victims, and all charred remains. It is up to the policies and procedures of the office who will interpret the resultant films and images; however, a forensic pathologist should feel comfortable with, and is totally capable of, interpretation of these images.

45

Evidence collection

In general there are four good rules of thumb with regard to evidence collection, which are (1) collect evidence in clearly labeled containers; (2) if the evidence must be stored, rather than receipted directly to law enforcement, store the evidence in a secure location; (3) document both photographically and in text; and (4) track everything with a chain of custody document.

In order to document contact between a suspect and decedent, samples will be taken from the decedent in order to assay for trace evidence or nucleic acid relationships. After documentation and photography of clothing "as is" on the body, trace evidence can be collected either by the forensic pathologist or by law enforcement who may be present during the autopsy. There may be institutional rules governing the presence of law enforcement in the autopsy suite during procurement of evidence, so they will have to be reviewed prior to evidence collection. In general, however, it is best practice for the forensic pathologist to identify, document, and have photographed any evidence *prior* to removal from the body. The pathologist will then procure the evidence using established technique(s) so as not to contaminate the evidence with extraneous material, and will use standard collection techniques (i.e., paper envelopes labeled with the case number, date collected; the type of contents; the name of the deceased; the name of the medical examiner or the responsible physician; and the name of the person securing the specimen) in order to procure specimens. In addition, following evidence procurement, it is good practice to photograph the evidence prior to final packaging with a scale containing the case number and then to package or cause packaging of the evidence immediately so that it is in its container, sealed with initialed evidence tape, and listed on an evidence receipt for submission to law enforcement or crime scene representatives. In order to ensure security of evidence, this writer will make sure that all evidence is packaged and documented on an evidence receipt *before* commencing any further in the external examination or autopsy. This limits the number of people who have "access" to the evidence and, as stated previously, makes the chain of custody as short as possible.

The type of evidence collected is case specific, although there are some useful generalities to commit to memory:

1. Fingernail swabs should be performed on all close-contact type homicides (i.e., stabbings, beatings, cervical compressions, etc.) and all suspicious deaths.

2. Physical evidence recovery (rape) kits should be used in *any* case where sexual contact is anticipated to have happened. This usually takes place when the decedent is found nude, partially clothed, with pants or pants and underwear pulled down, dresses or skirts pulled up, or when found in a sexually provocative position. Physical evidence recovery kits can be pre-formed by the local crime laboratory or can be assembled by the medical examiner/coroner's office themselves. In any case, the collection materials have to be clean, unopened, single use, well labeled, and well documented. If elements of the standard kit are not procured, a reason must be given so that it is not assumed that the particular element has simply been omitted (e.g., absence of hair if shaved or decedent not wearing underwear). A forensically sound rule of thumb is to visualize and photograph any surface or cavity *before* making contact with it with a swab or any other device (e.g., speculum in pelvic examinations). In this way, any true trauma can be delineated from postmortem artifact caused by the examiner. In general, the elements of the physical evidence recovery kit are the following:

A. Swabs of oral, vaginal (if female) or penile (if male), and rectal mucosae. The swabs can be smeared on a glass slide and the slides and swabs permitted to dry. Thereafter, the slides can be processed by staining with either hematoxylin–eosin or nuclear fast red and picroindigocarmine (Christmas tree stain) (if available). Any spermatozoa on the slide can be visualized by light microscopy and their presence may guide law enforcement investigative courses. Alternatively, the dried slides can be submitted to law enforcement to be examined by forensic laboratorians.

B. Pubic and scalp hair combings (using a clean single-use comb on a piece of clean single-use tissue paper and submission of the used comb folded and enclosed completely inside the tissue paper). Each should be packaged separately for obvious reasons.

C. Pubic and scalp hair exemplars, pulled by hand with root intact, and submitted in separate packages. The scalp hair exemplars, if possible and if the hair is available, will be pulled from the front, top, right, left, and back of the scalp in order to demonstrate all the different varieties of scalp hair of the decedent.

   D. Fingernail swabs with single-use sterile water, and/or fingernail clippings using sterile (bleached or isopropanol-cleaned) scissors or nail clippers.

   E. Any fibers/hair or loosely adherent material on the surface of the body or clothing. These can be picked up using standard techniques with appropriate collectors.

   F. The decedent's underwear, if present.

3. Clothing should be photographed and collected on all homicides, suspicious deaths, and all "hit and runs," in order to permit trace evidence documentation.

4. Scalp hair exemplars and all observed trace evidence should be collected from deaths that have occurred by suspected or witnessed "hit and runs."

5. The head should be shaved in cases of cephalic blunt force injury homicide or in any case where the pathologist must examine the head for patterned injuries on the scalp. All shaved hair should be saved for submission for trace evidence.

6. Any injuries considered to be a bitemark should be photographed with an American Board of Forensic Odontology (ABFO) scale, and swabbed for submission for nucleic acid studies. In addition, a Board-certified forensic odontologist (if available) should be called for consultation.

Autopsy

External examination

The normal procedure in most offices is that it is either the forensic pathologist's or the autopsy technician's duty to see that the body is prepared for autopsy, that the body is photographed "as is" or "dirty," and that any therapeutic devices are noted and recorded. Every autopsy should begin with a description of outside to in, and as such begins with the external examination. A body diagram or written list is utilized in order to document injuries, and marks of identification or therapeutic interventions. This kind of documentation permits the injuries to be qualified and at least partially quantified (at least in area) and to be "put in space"

on the decedent's body. Certain injuries are conventionally measured and documented from key anatomic references (e.g., gunshot and stab wounds are conventionally measured from the top of the head [above the waist] or sole of the ipsilateral foot [if below the waist], or ligature furrows on the neck from hangings are conventionally measured from the tip of the chin, the distance from each earlobe, and the ligature mark from the highest point on the body to the top of the head). Exit and entrance gunshot wounds, if known and determinable by morphologic examination, should be clearly marked for future reference.

Photographic documentation supports the textual descriptions in the autopsy report and establishes a visual record of the autopsy findings. Photos will be taken of all injuries, marks of therapy, and identifying marks. All photos should include both a distant, contextual photograph and a close-range photograph to demonstrate the details of the subject. In addition, all photos will contain a reference scale in at least one representation of injuries. At least one set of injury photographs will be unobstructed by blood, clothing, or foreign material.

In addition, all positive and negative findings will be documented photographically. Injuries are to be described by type (i.e., contusion, laceration, abrasion, gunshot wound of entry or of exit, stab wound, incised wound, etc.), by location (to be easily understood by a lay reader, but using proper medical terminology), by size (measured at least in greatest dimension), by shape and by pattern (e.g., stippled versus linear versus one with periodicity and areas of sparing), and if there are any associated injuries or patterns associated with the injuries listed (e.g., abrasions around a laceration or a series of linear or curvilinear red abrasions radiating from or adjacent to a stab wound suggesting the potential for a serrated stabbing instrument). This sort of documentation permits recall and description of injuries during court proceedings and also provides other pathologists who may be consulted for the case to make their own independent conclusions.

The body is then cleaned and all identifying marks, remote injuries, and any and all new injuries are noted and recorded and the body is re-photographed "clean." In some cases radiologic techniques are utilized to visualize evidence retained in the body, and the autopsy technician and/or forensic pathologist must be capable of not only operating an X-ray machine safely but also resolving the image either by standard chemical film processing or by digital image acquisition.

There are also numerous special procedures to be performed by the forensic pathologist, such as the sterile sampling of body fluid(s) for bacterial or viral culture, trace evidence collection in the form of alternative light examination of the body, clothing procurement and analysis for transfer-pattern recognition, trace evidence collection, fingernail and body-hair sampling for nucleic acid identity testing, or the sampling of fluids in the body cavities in search for evidence of sexual assault, all as previously described. Photographs may have to be taken following procurement of evidence at the discretion of the forensic pathologist.

Internal examination

The forensic pathologist, or autopsy technician under direct supervision by the forensic pathologist, then begins dissection of the body in an orderly manner, usually beginning with the standard "Y" incision from the anterior shoulders to the skin overlying the sternum or breastbone, which continues down the midline abdomen, around the umbilicus, and terminates at the pubic bone. This approach to opening the body enables visualization and access to the organs of the thorax, abdomen, and pelvis. Adhesions and fluids that are present in the body cavities (i.e., pleural, pericardial, or peritoneal) are noted and quantified for the final report. The organs will be inspected and examined *in situ* as well as following removal. It is before the removal of the organs that specimens for laboratory testing should be collected (see description below). Examination of the organs *in situ* provides the ability to document fluids collected in any occult spaces (ascites, hemopericardium, etc.), natural disease with all of the anatomic relationship preserved, as well as permitting the opportunity to document the details of tracks, direction, and depth of any injuries encountered. All the while, the forensic pathologist is examining the organs as they are removed, looking for natural diseases, traumatic injuries, and any evidence that may still be in the body (i.e., bullets, bullet jackets, or knife tips, etc.). Any abnormalities, injuries, or disease processes of interest are then photographed before they are removed. Organs can be removed by an assistant, but using best practice all organ removals should be directly observed by the pathologist of record. Following removal of the organs of the thorax, abdomen, and pelvis, attention is directed to the decedent's head where a coronal incision is made behind the ears and over the crown of the head. The scalp is peeled forward and backward from the incision and the pathologist inspects the underlying aponeurosis galea for contusions, hematomata, and associated trauma. After the scalp has been inspected, photographs may be taken to document findings (or lack of findings) of the top, front, and right and left sides of the scalp. Access to the brain and its coverings must be achieved. If the decedent is old enough for the fontanelles ("soft spots" of the top and back of the skull) to have fused, the brain is accessed by a vibratory saw. If the decedent is still an infant, the likelihood is high that the fontanelles have not yet fused and the brain can be accessed via incising the aponeurosis galea overlying the fontanelle and using scissors to cut down the unfused cranial sutures to the skull base. Upon opening, the pathologist inspects the dura and underlying brain and cerebellum for signs of infection (i.e., purulent exudate, vascular congestion, and dural or leptomeningeal erythema) or trauma (i.e., hematomata or hemorrhage in the potential space between the dura and the skull [epidural space], between the dura and the leptomeninges [subdural space], or between the leptomeninges and cerebral cortex proper [subarachnoid hemorrhage]). The brain and its coverings can be photographed in order to document the findings (or lack of findings), and then the pathologist or forensic technician will transect the medulla as it ramifies into the foramen magnum and will then remove the brain and cerebellum in one piece, careful to observe the base of the skull for occult hematomata or fluid collections. Once the brain and cerebellum have been removed, the dura of the skull base is removed in total in order for observation of the bones of the skull base in search for trauma (i.e., fractures in particular) or any natural disease states. Photographs can be taken at this stage in order to document the findings (or lack of findings), and once the pathologist is satisfied with the dissection, the cranium is put back together and the scalp is tacked closed with a stitch or two at the crown of the head. The organs that have been removed are then separated from each other (if removed *en bloc*), weighed (i.e., brain, heart, lungs, liver, kidneys, spleen, and, in children, the thymus and adrenals), are described grossly, photographed if needs be, and dissected further and serially sectioned by the forensic pathologist. During this phase, all of the tissue not saved by the pathologist for future study is deposited in a biohazard bag and the entire bag is transferred back into the body, and the body is sewn closed and cleaned again by the autopsy technician. In some cases, specialized dissections must be performed to give access to specific anatomic areas of organs (e.g., anterior neck dissections to assess trauma associated with cervical compression; posterior neck dissections to assess the cervical skeleton and spinal cord [to be done *after* removal of the brain and cerebellum], removal of the middle ear structures in order to observe inflammatory conditions and infections), or removal of the eyes in order to examine for retinal hemorrhages. In some cases the forensic pathologist may wish to hold the body for additional time in order to permit the vasculature of the skin to drain so that injuries, or injury patterns that are difficult to ascertain when congested with blood, can be resolved and documented more effectively.

The body is then prepared for transportation to the disposition of the family's choice (i.e., funeral home or crematorium). The autopsy is therefore often a "team event," in that there are at least two pairs of eyes on the body, organs, and the evidence.

The exemplar autopsy technician must be thoroughly trained in human anatomy, and is facile with even the most complex autopsy surgical procedures and wound assessment. It is the case in some offices that the autopsy technicians have either years of experience as anatomic prosectors either in academia or in hospital settings, or that they have experience as embalmers or funeral directors. The forensic pathologists must clearly be competent, observant, well trained, and meticulous. In either case, the team approach is consistently better and more efficient than any solo alternative. In addition, it must also be recognized that the pathology department not only functions to process the bodies, organs, and evidence in the autopsy suite, but also assures timely and efficient preparation of the body for the funeral homes and crematoria to which the bodies are transported in order for the families to be able to make their final plans.

Specimens for laboratory testing

Specimens for laboratory testing will be collected in almost every case that is accessioned; the exceptions would be skeletons or bodies that are so decomposed (i.e., putrified or mummified) that there are no body fluids remaining in the body.

An important rule of thumb for important information to discover before collection of decedent blood for assay (i.e., toxicology, nucleic acid-based identification, metabolic panels for inborn errors of metabolism, etc.) is to find out: (1) if the decedent has had a blood or blood product transfusion; and (2) if the decedent has been transfused, that any/all testing will be performed on a sample of decedent pre-transfusion blood. Thus if the decedent were transported to the hospital, the death investigator will have to find out the transfusion status of the decedent in order to make this ascertainment. If the decedent was transfused, the death investigator can make contact with the hospital laboratory's "central receiving" and/or the hospital blood bank, both of which are great resources for decedent blood that has been drawn while in the hospital. The samples can be transported securely with the body or can be picked up by the death investigator or law enforcement personnel separate from transport.

Toxicology testing

There are certain samples that are routinely collected and, as they are considered to be evidence, these have to be properly labeled and packaged in a conventional manner. The manner in which samples are collected will be in agreement with good laboratory practices and the vessels in which the samples are collected and stored must be appropriate for the sample and testing modalities ordered. Strict adherence to good laboratory practice and the directives of the toxicology staff of the office or that laboratory contracted by the office will ensure that the results of the testing will be valid and useful. Typical samples, if available, collected from non-decomposed decedents are the following:

1. blood
2. urine
3. vitreous fluid
4. bile.

Some office policies are that organ tissue is also collected for testing, or at least stored for potential testing later. In general, sections of liver, brain, and sometimes kidney, and all gastric contents, are stored for potential testing later. When considering what blood vessels to sample, peripheral blood (i.e., subclavian, femoral, or iliac) is preferable to central blood (i.e., heart, portal, or caval sources) because of the concept of postmortem redistribution and the anatomy of the enterohepatic circulation, which is exhaustively covered elsewhere. In some cases there will not be choices for blood sampling as the decedent may have hemorrhaged after injury and there may be little intravascular blood present. The blood present following injury may have collected in the pericardial sac, the pleural spaces, or the peritoneal space, thus that will have to be collected. In any case, the source of the blood

49

(i.e., heart, central, peripheral, cavity, subdural, etc.) will be labeled on the sample once collected and the sample will be submitted to the laboratory in a package that is sealed, well labeled with the case number and the date collected; the type of contents; the name of the deceased; the name of the medical examiner or the responsible physician; and the name of the person securing the specimen. The samples will be accompanied by an evidence receipt in order to document the chain of custody for the laboratory or laboratory agent.

Histologic examination

In general, tissues for histologic examination are taken at the discretion of the pathologist. This discretion is developed by practice habits, office funding, and the experience of the practitioner. Thus forensic pathologists have a non-uniform approach to histology. It is forensically prudent to store formalinized tissue sections in some fashion for a reasonable time period (one to two years, depending on jurisdictional rules or statute) on every case if histologic examination becomes warranted later; however, it is not necessary to put histology through on every case. In any case, where an anatomic cause of death is not appreciated or determined at autopsy, putting histologic sections through may be a good idea in order to examine for microscopic evidence of lethal disease and/or microscopic evidence of the sequelae of trauma while other assays are being performed (i.e., toxicology, cultures, etc.). NAME directs pathologists to perform histological examinations in cases with no gross anatomic cause of death unless the remains are skeletonized. Additionally, it is prudent and is compulsory in some jurisdictions to take tissue samples in cases of infant death to include, but not limited to: cerebrum, midbrain, cerebellum, cervical spinal cord, heart, lungs, thyroid gland, liver, kidneys, adrenal glands, spleen, thymus, esophagus, stomach, small intestine, large intestine, rectum, gonads, prostate and urinary bladder (males), and vagina/cervix (females). Other sections that may be useful, especially in infant deaths, are cerebral white matter tracts (i.e., corpus callosum, internal capsule, pons, medulla; the entire pons/medulla/cervical spine) for examination of any diffuse axonal injury; generous leptomeningeal membrane sampling for examination of occult inflammation; longitudinal section through tongue, epiglottis, larynx, and trachea to examine for occult upper airway inflammation; and transverse sectioning through mid-trachea and esophagus at the level of the thyroid gland in order to examine the entire foregut, thyroid, and any associated parathyroid tissue in a single, efficient section.

Metabolic panels

These are generally pre-formed test cards constructed of filter paper, property receipt, and areas to record demographic information. Decedent blood is spotted on the filter paper and, once dried, the sample is sent to a laboratory for assay. Typical metabolic panels assay for congenital adrenal hyperplasia (CAH), congenital hypothyroidism, galactosemia, and glucose-6-phosphate dehydrogenase (G6PD) deficiency. Further blood samples can be taken (in the appropriate tube) for testing for hemoglobinopathies and other inborn errors. In this age, most of this testing is compulsory for newborns in the hospital by statute, thus the data for these assays are searchable and able to be requested with medical records from the birth hospital. However, if this information is not available because it cannot be found or verified personally by the forensic pathologist, the decedent's blood can be easily assayed if a metabolic disorder is considered material to the death. If the decedent has a state metabolic panel on file, a new metabolic profile is generally not necessary.

Microbiology testing

This modality of testing is under the discretion of the forensic pathologist and is based on their experience and training. In some cases microbiological testing is completely irrelevant and in others it is the crux of the cause and manner certification of the case. In general, there is an inverse relationship between postmortem interval and validity of postmortem microbiology, thus as the postmortem interval increases the utility and validity of postmortem cultures decrease. In general the sooner microbiological samples can be procured the more valid the samples will be; thus if infection is considered to be in the differential diagnosis for cause of death, then cultures should be collected as soon as is possible. If the decedent has been transported to, or admitted into, the hospital, the hospital may have collected and submitted cultures they drew under sterile conditions. If this is the case, the hospital should be contacted to continue monitoring the cultures for the typical time period (usually five days). If samples have been collected from the decedent at the hospital, but not submitted to the laboratory, the hospital lab can be asked by the forensic pathologist to run the samples to completion *or*, alternatively, the samples can be transported to the office with the body and other samples and the forensic pathologist can submit the cultures to their contracted laboratory (if the laboratory can process those sample containers [there are several different types]). If no samples have been collected and the postmortem interval is reasonable (a reasonable margin for validity of results is less than 24 hours in our experience), microbiological samples can be collected in the morgue as part of the autopsy. Appropriate mechanisms of sterilization should be employed (i.e., cautery, betadine, or iso-propanol) and samples can be collected into appropriately labeled tubes, vessels, or culturettes. Typical samples include but are not limited to blood for bacterial cultures, lung and spleen tissue or culturette swab for bacterial cultures, cerebral spinal fluid (CSF) for bacterial cultures, a leptomeningeal culturette swab for bacterial cultures, and a nasopharyngeal swab placed in viral transport medium for respiratory virus cultures. Certainly if there is any gross evidence of infection or inflammation (i.e., abscesses, exudates, sinus tracts, fistulae, etc.) separate from the aforementioned collections, these should be both cultured and submitted for histological examination.

Post-autopsy processes and procedures

To pend or certify?

Certification of death, to a certain extent, is based on the experience and training of the forensic pathologist as well as the culture of the office in question. In general, if the cause and manner of death are grossly demonstrable or historically documented within a reasonable degree of medical certainty by the completion of autopsy or external examination, it is appropriate to certify the cause and manner at that time. If the cause and manner are anatomically, circumstantially, or historically unclear in any fashion or by any means, the certification should be pending further investigation. If there is further investigation required by *any* agency, the certification should be pending the satisfactory completion of that/those investigations. In addition, if the results of any laboratory testing (i.e., histology, toxicology, microbiology, metabolic panel) or consultancy are being considered material to proper death certification, the certification should be pending the completion of those studies and review of those results.

Evidence disposition

It is most forensically prudent to submit evidence to law enforcement as soon as possible during or after the examination of the body (i.e., external examination or autopsy). In general, offices of medical examiners and coroners are not as secure as those of law enforcement and, as such, any storage of evidence by non-law enforcement associated offices is fraught with potential problems and insecurity. If evidence is not taken during or directly following examination, an agreement should be struck with law enforcement personnel that evidence will be picked up within a reasonable and mutually agreed upon time period (48 to 72 hours). This agreement should be developed into a signed policy and procedure for all material law enforcement agencies and the death investigatory office. In addition, the medical examiner/coroner's office should have in place a mechanism in order to inform law enforcement of the storage of evidence and that it will be disposed of after the time limit of evidence holding for that jurisdiction has been met. These rules of evidence retention are often described or promulgated in statute or by judicial administrative order. The death investigators and forensic pathologists should be aware of these retention orders and should educate law enforcement of these rules as well, where applicable. Thus law enforcement personnel are made aware of retained evidence and that they have, for example, a year from the date of the autopsy to collect the evidence or it will be appropriately disposed of as provided by statute or administrative order. An effective and legally responsible means of this notice is by certified letter to the detective of record such that a signature is rendered to the office of medical examiner/coroner as proof of receipt of the information on disposition. The receipt should be made part of the case for later reference.

The office of medical examiner or coroner *must* be aware of the statutory obligations they have with regard to evidence and should stringently adhere to those obligations. At the exception of statutory or judicial order obligation, offices *should not* be made to feel as though they *have* to store said evidence past the obligatory time period provided in statute, and nor should they feel as though they should store it willingly. There must be a resonance with the law enforcement agencies of record, and it is this writer's experience that as long as all policies and procedures are stringently adhered to on a consistent basis, there are few issues that arise. This is not to say that all evidence must be disposed of or destroyed, or on a schedule for disposal or destruction. There is some evidence that may be important for casework, which the forensic pathologist, medical examiner, or coroner wishes to be saved for future legal actions, thus there must be a mechanism in place to track these items by evidence receipt.

In addition, there must be a mechanism in place for outside agents (e.g., families and attorneys) to request the saving and maintenance of evidence and have their requests be honored. These request are best limited by time (i.e., once requested, a certified letter is sent to the requestor directing them that they have three to six, or twelve, months to have the item(s) assessed by an expert or otherwise impounded) and that after the allotted time period, the evidence will be appropriately disposed of or destroyed.

Regular disposal and destruction of surplus evidentiary material, after the statutorily provided obligatory time period, is part and parcel of the operations of these offices as laboratories and proper procedures and documentation should be created and be in place to capture these regular activities.

Toxicology assay versus holding toxicology

A general rule of thumb is that if there is no apparent anatomic cause of death ascertained during autopsy, toxicological testing should be performed in order to rule out death caused by or contributed to by intoxication. This is especially true in cases of death in children, as occult or clandestine poisonings are possible and may not be revealed by interviewing caregivers or family members. There are many ways caregivers or family members may inadvertently (e.g., ethanol or aspirin used to soothe sore gums during teething, or diphenhydramine in order to sedate a colicky infant) or even purposefully intoxicate a child. In addition, as children get older and are able to "cruise" or walk around on their own, anything within reach is likely to go near or in their mouths, to which all parents and anyone who has ever taken care of an infant can attest. Thus medications or drugs or paraphernalia left on sitting surfaces, between couch or chair cushions, on coffee tables or end tables, lying on the floor after falling from someone's pocket all are now in hands' reach of the infant or toddler. This being the case, deaths with no anatomic cause at autopsy must be assayed for intoxicating substances. It is generally best to have a standard approach to toxicology where drug screens for large drug groups (opiates, benzodiazepines, barbiturates, amphetamines, xanthines [caffeine and acetaminophen or Tylenol], salicylates, etc.) are performed on the urine and if any of them are positive, then further, more directed, testing is performed on the blood. Infants and toddlers may have little to no urine stored in their urinary bladder upon autopsy because, developmentally, they are still working on conscious control of their urinary habits and are likely wearing diapers, "pull ups," or some other absorbent undergarment. In these cases, it is forensically prudent to impound the absorbent undergarment and submit it as evidence to toxicology for potential testing later if needs be. In cases with no urine, toxicology screens can be performed on the blood samples. Interpretation of toxicology results in infants is also difficult because, both thankfully and sadly, there are limited data on lethal and toxic levels of many medications and illicit substances in infants and children. This being the case, at the exclusion of any other gross or microscopic anatomic cause of death and full investigation, considerable attention must be given to any substance(s) detected in the infant or child blood samples. Positive toxicology results in the infant or child samples should prompt further investigation into the medicament list of the decedent as well as the behaviors of the caregiver(s) or family members and whether there is any connection between what was found in the decedent's samples and drugs/medications used by caregiver(s)/family members. In addition, the finding of medications and substances not typically prescribed or indicated for infants or children (e.g., methadone) should prompt further investigation, regardless of the level in the decedent's plasma. It is in these cases that careful interviewing of the parent(s)/caregiver(s) can yield potentially useful information regarding cause and manner of death. Because the finding of potentially intoxicating substances in the samples from an infant or child can lead to a criminal investigation, it is at this time that law enforcement should be engaged in order to permit them to either: (1) take over the investigation; or (2) at least take part in all questioning of the family member(s)/caregiver(s) so that all of the responses given to questions are heard and documented by law enforcement personnel. In general, it is the experience of these writers that some law enforcement agents either are recalcitrant to believe that parent(s)/caregiver(s) may be responsible for lethal intoxication of their child or they have difficulty engaging in these types of investigations because it is not a straight criminal *or* death investigation. These cases are often also made more difficult when parent(s)/caregiver(s) are considered to be potentially culpable (either accidentally or purposefully) for the death of a child, there is then a question of engaging other investigative agencies (i.e., child protective services) and/or removal of any other children from the household for their own protection. It is important for the death investigation agency to remain clinical and objective with regard to their findings and opinions. Without parent or caregiver admission of actively "feeding" or administering the child an intoxicating substance, all that can be said about such findings is that the substance(s) was/were found in the sample(s) taken at autopsy. Based on the sites where the samples were found (i.e., peripheral blood, bile, or gastric), routes of administration and acuteness or chronicity of administration can be opined, but a defensible opinion of circumstances may not be able to be ascertained or offered. Again, a tremendous amount of humility and care must be given when rendering these opinions and the more objective (and therefore defensible) the opinion, the better.

Identification

NAME Autopsy Performance Standards direct that identification methods include viewing the remains either in person or by photograph (where the decedent is identified by case number) by contacts who have known the decedent in life; by comparison of antemortem exemplar and postmortem dental imaging/charts, fingerprints or body radiographs; or by nucleic acid profile comparison with a known exemplar from the decedent or comparison to nucleic acid sampled from a first-order relative. Therefore in every case the death investigator and pathologist should assure the sufficiency of presumptive identification, will photograph and document the clothing and personal effects, and will either take themselves or direct the photography of the decedent regarding any marks of identification of the decedent (i.e., moles, tattoos, scars, marks of therapy, or congenital/acquired idiosyncratic anatomic abnormalities) with appropriate case identifiers, and should document, procure, and properly store nucleic acid samples for the obligatory time period in the prescribed fashion. Any unidentified or presumptively identified decedent should undergo whole body radiography not only in order to search for injuries or evidence retained in the body (e.g., projectiles or knife tips), but also the presence of surgical devices, and stigmata of previous medical or dental interventions (e.g., prosthetic joints, pacemakers, dental amalgams or prostheses).

In cases of unidentified or presumptively identified infants or children, an autopsy will be most likely performed because of the lack of known past medical history. As with any unidentified body, it is important to understand that autopsy is useful not only in determination of cause of death, but also can disclose the presence of medical conditions or surgical appliances that may be useful in identification. The teeth of the decedent should also be radiographed in the standard way using conventionally accepted odontological procedures, and the dentition of the unidentified or presumptively identified decedent will be charted by either a forensic pathologist or forensic odontologist, and the death investigator should be directed to begin searching for exemplar antemortem dental records on the presumed person, should they exist. In children, the parents may or may not have taken the child to the dentist prior to the child's death. Infants almost *never* have had any dental interventions unless there was a skeletal abnormality of the maxilla or mandible. Thus the presence of antemortem dental records is completely unpredictable and likely uncommon, depending on the age of the child. Assurance of proper initial documentation can avoid the need for subsequent exhumation in the future.

Consultation

The need for consultation depends solely on the forensic pathologist, their skill set, experience, training, physical and financial access to consultants, and the policies and procedures of their office. Photographs of the fresh organ(s) or tissue(s) of interest should be taken and the organ or tissue can be saved in formalin until the consultant can arrive for their examination. Upon arrival of the consultant, the case history, hospital findings (if any), photographs, and preliminary autopsy findings should be made available so that they are fully aware of all pertinent findings to date. Alternatively, the forensic pathologist may feel comfortable enough with the gross and microscopic findings that they consider consultancy to be redundant and not additive to the case. This is an important consideration, especially as forensic pathologists are the steward of public funding and, as such, must be deliberate in their expenditures and spending habits. Other offices may require consultant services in certain cases (e.g., neuropathology consultant examination in every case of lethal injury to the head of all causes – gunshots, blunt force, sharp force, etc.). Neither is correct or incorrect and neither must be compared as every system operates differently, as previously discussed.

Case consultation by experts in the field (i.e., pediatric cardiologists or electrophysiologists, neuropathologists, cardiac pathologists, etc.) should be utilized liberally as their opinion(s) are useful for confirming the impressions of the forensic pathologist, to guide the pathologist as to directions and avenues for study or testing, and to lend credence on opinions and certifications. It is important to remember that the forensic pathologist reviews all histology, tissues, dissections, and reports submitted by consultants in order to attain comprehensive understanding of the case. In addition, it is the forensic pathologist's case – *not* that of the consultant, thus the pathologist of record must incorporate the findings into their final autopsy report and must be responsible for all findings reported. The best way to lose consultants is to get them entangled in testimony regarding their opinions. Consultants offer an opinion and the pathologist can seek to use the information or not depending on its merit and the *pathologist* is *solely responsible* for the content of their reports and should be the witness to deliver case findings listed in the final report, not the consultant.

When consulting, it is prudent to make sure your consultant has all the relevant investigative, historical, laboratory, and medical information known to date – to include the preliminary autopsy findings, access to all autopsy photographs, any laboratory testing pending or complete, medical records, and any/all associated histologic findings. The more informed they are, the better they can tailor their consultation. If the consultant will perform their examination in your presence and permit photo-documentation or if their slide reading can be performed with you present, it has been this writer's experience that the consultation is also better informed and you can ask and answer questions in real time.

Additional information needed after autopsy

Cases of infant or child death can be confusing at times because of numerous caregivers, the vagaries of growth and development, and relatives who have interests in finding the cause and manner of death and who may offer misinformation or even disinformation during the investigation.

If the decedent were transported to, or admitted into, the hospital where death was pronounced, a medical record will be requested to accompany the body when transported to the office for examination.

Following external, or autopsy, examination more medical records may be required in order to better assess the decedent's antemortem state of health and past medical/surgical histories. In most cases, the medical record(s) will be short because the infant/child has only been on the planet a short while (less than 18 years) and, as such, likely has not seen the doctor or been hospitalized too many times. The records requested will depend on not only the age of the decedent, but also the nature and circumstances of the case. For instance, in cases where an infant or child has sustained anatomically demonstrable multiple blunt force injuries in a motor vehicle crash, there is no need to request previous medical records as the cause is patently obvious and is not attributable to anything in the medical record. In cases of infant/child death where there is no anatomically demonstrable cause of death at autopsy, medical records should be requested *pro forma*.

In cases of infant death with no anatomically demonstrable cause of death, the records requested should include records of maternal pregnancy, all birth records, to include delivery and neonatal intensive care unit (NICU) admission(s) (if any), state metabolic disease panel and discharge summary, all pediatric well baby and sick visits (as appropriate), and all hospital admissions or emergency department visits up to the date of death. In the cases of infants who were taken to the hospital and had any subsequent treatment leading up to death, all those records including the EMS run-sheet should be requested.

In cases of the death of an older child, depending on the age of the child and the circumstances of the case, death investigators may choose medical records from closer to the time of death in order to discern any sentinel events that may have heralded the death, rather than illogically collecting birth records on a 16-year-old child who appears, by investigation, to have overdosed on heroin. In addition, older children may have seen therapists or specialists about certain problems and requesting those records may be helpful in direction for cause of death determination.

Law enforcement follow-up

If law enforcement is present for the autopsy, they will naturally be updated as the case proceeds. If injuries suspicious for criminality are appreciated during autopsy, law enforcement will have to begin their potential criminal death investigation and will have to be educated and coached as to the kinds of injuries that were found and what may have caused them (if that can be determined or opined to a reasonable degree of medical certainty). Depending on their level of experience and training, law enforcement personnel may also have to be coached and educated as to the questions to ask the parent(s)/caregiver(s) in order not to imply or lead too much, and still elicit as much information as they can. Skilled law enforcement agents are expert at gaining trust of and interviewing witnesses. In fact, all transcripts and video documentation of subsequent interviews should be reviewed by the forensic pathologist for correlation to the anatomic and laboratory findings.

If no injuries suspicious for criminality are discovered at autopsy and ancillary laboratory tests and histologic examination is pending, law enforcement should be briefed on the findings to date and that other tests are pending. If a non-natural death is being entertained due to anatomic findings and/or scene findings, medical records, or investigatory information, law enforcement should be informed of the weight that each of the sources of information is being given and whether the results of laboratory testing (i.e., toxicology, histology, microbiology, metabolic panels, etc.) are material to the death and, if so, that the case will be pended until those data are made available.

In cases where law enforcement is not present at the autopsy, if inexplicable, or lethal, injuries are discovered during autopsy, the lead detective(s) should be called and their presence requested for the remainder of the autopsy, which may be paused for their arrival. It may be that there was no indication of foul play or trauma upon initial scene assessment by both law enforcement and death investigators and their attention may have been drawn away from this case by other, pressing matters or mitigating factors. Thus the findings of injuries may be a complete surprise to law enforcement and their presence for the remainder of the autopsy may alter the course of their investigation. In general, the sooner one can engage law enforcement, the better. Early involvement of law enforcement gives them time to collect as much information as they can as early as possible, permitting detectives to lock witnesses into sworn, taped statements with which further autopsy findings may be correlated.

If law enforcement is not present and no anatomic cause of death is appreciated during autopsy, law enforcement should be contacted soon after finishing the autopsy and the case findings (or lack of findings) discussed. The case should be pended upon review of the decedent's medical records and for the remaining ancillary testing to be performed and any subsequent data reviewed.

Discussion with parents/caregivers?

This is a decision based upon the case findings at autopsy.

If there are *no* findings at autopsy and the case is pending ancillary laboratory testing as well as review of the medical records, the parent(s)/caregiver(s) should be contacted and the findings conveyed to them. The discussion should be for a lay audience and should essentially take the form that no anatomic cause of death was appreciated (i.e., injuries, signs of infection, cancer, metabolic problems, or anatomic abnormalities), that the medical records will be requested and reviewed, and that results from other testing are pending. At this time, further discussion of the decedent's medical history as well as family history can be made in order to get a better sense as to the decedent's previous state of health. In addition, if it has not been performed already, the benefits of a reconstruction may be discussed (if the decedent is an infant, or an older child, and there is any thought that a reconstruction may assist with the determination of cause and manner of death). The parent(s)/caregiver(s) should also be told that law enforcement will be included in any reconstruction so that it would not have to be repeated, and so that all material agencies have all of the information possible. An approximate time frame (where possible) of the final results to be received should be given to the parent(s)/caregiver(s) and they should be given your contact information for any further questions or information they may have.

It is this writer's experience that filtering all case facts through the appointed law enforcement agent (usually a detective) is the most prudent approach to death cases. By doing so, the forensic pathologist (1) permits law enforcement to have an opinion on information dispersal; and (2) there is relative assurance that since law enforcement has been given the opportunity to filter case information, there will be the avoidance of problems down the road.

Though arguable and completely idiosyncratic per the forensic pathologist, medical examiner, or coroner involved, if there are findings worrisome for criminality or just suspicious for the time being, it is advisable that very limited discussion should be initiated with the parent(s)/caregiver(s) in favor of law enforcement being the spokesperson, so that all information is filtered through law enforcement in the interests of any criminal case being developed. Any thoughts of discussion with the parent(s)/caregiver(s) should likely first be discussed with law enforcement in order to establish how the investigation will proceed and to prevent any miscommunication among involved parties. The idea is to not bias the testimony of the parent(s)/caregiver(s) or the view of antemortem events. The inclusion of law enforcement in these decisions also provides them with the ability to have more information than any potential suspects, for the purposes of their investigation and potential criminal case.

If the anatomic or historical findings are non-natural, but do not immediately rise to the level of criminality or criminal suspicion (e.g., drowning, near drowning, suffocation, suicide, or accidental trauma), the findings should still be filtered through law enforcement prior to discussion with the parent(s)/caregiver(s) in order to avoid inadvertently interfering with a criminal investigation by the discussion of findings. In these cases, the findings should be discussed as succinctly and clinically as possible without unnecessary description or detail in order not to upset or inflame an already tragic situation.

In any case, when parent(s)/family/caregiver(s) are contacted in the absence of an active criminal investigation, the death investigator/forensic pathologist should also convey to them the history/circumstances known to date in order to check the validity of the information and to permit them to amend, supplement, or clarify any details that may not have been made clear, were omitted, are erroneous, or which may not have been known at the time the original circumstances were investigated. In addition, as time passes and discussions are had between witnesses, family members, or caregivers, material information can be uncovered and added to the case. Also, time may give the witnesses, family members, or caregivers an opportunity to find or uncover details or further information that was not initially known as they clean, move, and store the decedent's property after the death. Thus intermittent contact should be made with witnesses, family members, or caregivers over the days and weeks subsequent to the autopsy in order to recalibrate the investigation and update the case information.

Autopsy report

There are many different formats for autopsy reports but, in general, an autopsy report should contain historic, gross, microscopic, and laboratory findings, which are described in sufficient detail to support the certification, diagnoses, and opinions rendered. Manner of death, depending on the jurisdiction, may be included or not, as it is merely an opinion based upon the circumstances known at the time of certification and is philosophically refutable and potentially contentious by its very nature. Opinions, their references, and any supporting documentation should be isolated from the objective portion of the report, which should have its own section. As such, the objective gross and microscopic findings should not contain opinions as to "large" or "small," but should be measured in two or three dimensions and reported as such.

Quality control processes

Quality control for reports of autopsy and external exams is important for consistency, readability, precision, as an internal control for training purposes, and in order to keep causes and manners of death reasonable and defensible. Offices use various quality control mechanisms to achieve their goals and adhere to NAME guidelines in their accreditation checklist. The NAME accreditation checklist advises that offices should have a written and implemented policy covering and directing quality control procedures. The quality control program should include a feedback procedure so that errors or findings that require clarification are brought to the attention of the pathologist of record. The quality control program should be planned and regularly scheduled and should be adequate enough to assure the quality of the office or system work products. There should be documentation of the corrective actions, if any, taken for deficiencies that are identified. Finally, the office should have a mechanism in place in order to track overdue case reports (NAME requires 90% of cases to be completed within 90 calendar days and suggests that 90% of autopsy cases should be completed within 60 calendar days). As an additional measure, it is good practice to review cases that have been judged not to reach jurisdictional criteria. This "turn down" review should occur the day following the cases having been called in so that if the cases have to be reviewed and potentially accepted later, the decedents have not been transported out of the office's jurisdiction, cremated, or buried, and so that the family is not unduly inconvenienced. There are some jurisdictions in which this review must be completed and documented within 24 hours of the death call. Offices have various triggers for their quality control review. Some offices will review every ten or twenty cases, others will review every case. In addition, offices may also procedurally require the Chief Medical Examiner or their proxy to *review* and *co-sign* every certified homicide in order to assure the quality of the investigation, and to review report consistency and completeness of injury descriptions.

Typical questions asked of reviewers on quality control reports are:

1. Are the demographics correct?
2. Does the cause of death make sense?
3. Is the investigation complete enough to support the cause and manner of death?
4. Are rights and lefts correct?
5. Are the descriptions complete enough that photographs are not required to understand the injuries?
6. Is the histologic examination complete and interpreted correctly?
7. Is the toxicology interpreted correctly?
8. Are there any typos?
9. Is the file complete?

In order to perform the review, the reviewing pathologist should have access to the entire case file, the "complete" autopsy report, toxicology (if any), histologic slides (if any), and autopsy photos.

Once finished, the reviewing pathologist should return the case materials to the pathologist of record and be available for discussion of the findings/issues (if any) so that there is agreement or at least some defensible reasoning established between them. Disagreements that cannot be resolved between the two can either be mitigated by the Chief Medical Examiner or their proxy, or the case could be brought before the pathologists in the group as a learning and case-review exercise. Pathologists should be comfortable enough to be critiqued and not become upset or resentful. The issue is that any problems should be mitigated and agreed upon before the case is signed out and released for public consumption.

Pending cases

As previously mentioned, the act of pending a case is idiosyncratic for each practicing pathologist and is

based on good practice, their level of experience, their type of training, their acceptance of the case information, and trust in the abilities of the death investigators and law enforcement agents. If there are any questions regarding the case information, the medical record, the injuries, the laboratory testing, or the circumstances, the most prudent course of action is to pend the certification of the case and engage the processes required to answer the questions or clarify the ambiguous.

Information commonly needed for certification

As intimated and stated explicitly in previous sections, types of information required to answer clinical or investigatory questions are myriad, protean, and case dependent. They can range from just being able to ask the detective some simple questions about patterns found on the body, to requiring a full criminal investigation of the scene, witnesses, and circumstances, with scene reconstruction or post-autopsy scene analysis. Commonly, cases are pending for some further information from family, law enforcement, medical professionals who cared for the decedent in life, or just to receive and review medical records. A common group of records required for pending cases is:

1. Admission history and physicals
2. Progress notes
3. Consultation notes
4. EMS runsheets
5. Operative notes
6. Imaging studies (i.e., tomographic or CT scans, magnetic resonance images or MRIs, radiographs or X-rays, or sometimes other types depending on the case)
7. Laboratory results.

Please note that depending on the case and its course, the records that may be required may be from various and non-continuous time periods, so the medicolegal death investigator is going to have to be clear on what to request, and the forensic pathologist, medical examiner, or coroner should have reviewed the case such that they are requesting the records from the material time periods.

Medical records from most hospitals these days are available electronically (usually as PDF documents) and, as such, will be received much faster than those sent via regular mail. Certain primary care physician offices, smaller hospital systems, nursing homes, and, occasionally, hospice systems may still utilize paper records, but these can be scanned on site and sent via facsimile or via email as a PDF document. These documents may take more time, as it takes clerical staff time to parse through the record and send what was requested versus reflexively sending the entire medical record.

The death investigatory office must then be able to store these records in some form. If the office can only store electronic records, the paper records (or the material portions of the records) can be scanned and saved electronically in a file on the office computer system, or in the electronic "file," or laboratory information management system (LIMS) – a paperless *Nirvana* to which many offices now aspire. If the office can only store paper records (which is a rarity in these days of inexpensive scanners and ubiquitous computer systems), then the medical records should be stored in a file physically linked to the case file and should follow the case file through all of its movements from office to storage. This writer has found it advantageous to notate the medical records that are crucial in opinions rendered about the case in various ways. These notated records can then be scanned and made part of the electronic record or electronic file, so that if the file is ever reviewed by another pathologist or consultant, they will be made fully aware of the reasons for certain opinions and have a clear clinical or investigational referent by which to render their own opinions or use as a source of further investigation.

The importance of requesting records from specific time periods of interest cannot be underscored enough. Much time can be wasted requesting or reading records from non-essential or immaterial time periods. In addition, the requesting pathologist and requestors must be clear about the source of the records, as there may be several hospital systems in a particular jurisdiction and records from the immaterial hospital system are not helpful to the case. If the hospital system of interest is not known, a "shotgun" approach can be taken by the requestor wherein a request is made using the decedent's name from the largest hospital systems in the area first to see what is available and then to hone the search later. If this does not bear fruit, a request can be made to hospital systems near the decedent's residence as people tend to stay "local" with regard to healthcare. Also, if the decedent were "at large" or did not have a

permanent residence, medical record requests to free clinics and community medical clinics can be made. If none of this works, the family, friends, or associates can be contacted in order to see if the decedent ever told them that they went to see a doctor anywhere.

If the decedent had a residence and it is still available to the death investigatory office, the police or legally authorized person can accompany staff to the decedent's residence in order to look for medication bottles, business cards, or any loose paperwork that may have a physician's name on it. There are times when the medicolegal staff must spend a great deal of time sifting through personal belongings in order to determine whether a decedent had a physician, for medical records, or a dentist, for dental record exemplars for scientific identification. Some cases are not straightforward in the least and the death investigators must have the resources and wherewithal to stay the course in looking for needed information. For infants and children this is much less common – as nearly all have seen physicians with relative frequency as infants require their well visits and vaccinations, and older children are required by schools to have periodic physicals and vaccine boosters. Thus infants and children are far better medically "characterized" and "documented" than some adults.

How to request information and from whom

The office should have mechanisms in place for information requests in all forms. Office clerical assistants can handle simple record requests and make appointments for scene reviews; however, well-trained medicolegal death investigators are the best sources of investigatory information due to their unique training and understanding of the processes of death certification. This writer has experienced several investigatory departments who have excellent relations with law enforcement and have the forensic and medical skillset to discuss case details with family, medical personnel, and law enforcement. There is no replacement, however, for forensic pathologists talking to material witnesses, law enforcement, family members, and medical personnel themselves. The pathologist of record should know everything about the cases and is the sole source for and interpreter of questions and answers, respectively. In addition, it often takes less time for the pathologist to get on the phone and resolve issues than to have an intermediary going "back and forth" between information sources and the pathologist.

Incorporation of consultant reports and their findings

The consultancy used for assistance as subject matter expertise can take a couple of forms. The consultant can review the case or subject matter of the case and give you an "unofficial" opinion, which is colloquially called a "curbside consult." These are used widely in order to verify or refute a pathologist's findings and provide a good checking mechanism before rendering an official opinion on a case. These largely go unnoticed as they are simply unofficial opinions by colleagues used to gauge and temper the opinion and interpretations of the pathologist of record.

The other type of consult, the official consult, is one in which the consultant renders a report that is made part of the case file. The pathologist of record must always review the same information and subject matter as the consultant in order to form their own opinion. When the pathologist has finished their review, if they agree, the findings are made part of the autopsy report. The opinion in the final anatomic diagnosis will be the pathologist's own, but will be indicated specially and will likely be referred back to the consultant's report (e.g., "see the outside cardiovascular pathology report"). In this way, anyone reading the final report will know that there is a consultant's report available, which can be requested for review or at least used as a referent as needed. Some jurisdictions have open public record laws where any document not under active investigation is open for "discovery" by any public figure – whether they have a material interest in the case or case information or not. Other jurisdictions do not have open public record laws, and the public have no material right to any documents that the office does not wish to tender them. Thus, this is another reason to be familiar with the statutes of the jurisdiction in which one works so as not to transgress by being either too open or not open enough with the availability of documents. The corollary to this is that staff in these offices must take care to know what is in the file, and that whatever is there must be defensible and well documented. This writer has had autopsy reports placed as PDF documents on media websites minutes after finalization, thus the appropriateness and precision of the verbiage used in these reports is crucial because they can quickly be consumed by the public.

Laboratory results

Laboratory results can be reported in the final anatomic diagnosis (though they are not in and of themselves "anatomic"). In fact, if the cause of death is demonstrated through a laboratory test (e.g., toxicology) it may even be the first item on the list. There will be autopsy protocol "purists" who will hold that the final anatomic diagnosis is for anatomic findings only. It is this writer's belief that in order for the autopsy report to read appropriately and to be clear and concise, an orderly process of listing trauma, toxicologic, and natural disease processes must be achieved in the autopsy report. That having been said, a rank order lists from most lethal, or what would be considered the cause of death, down to mundane findings such as "minor scattered contusions" or "remote cholecystectomy." It is important to list all of the different testing performed so that a reader is aware of what was completed and their contributions (if any) in the processes of cause and manner of death certification. The most effective way this writer has seen this be achieved is on the final anatomic diagnosis. Thus if a laboratory test was performed it is listed followed by the results. If the results did not add anything to the case, an interpretation of "non-contributory" can be listed to indicate that the results of that testing were not additive to the certification of the case. If the results of the testing are material to the cause and manner of death (e.g., cases of bacterial infection; drug intoxication; or hyperglycemia, metabolic acidosis, and ketosis, which indicate diabetic ketoacidosis), then the "diagnosis" listed as the cause of death (e.g., acute cocaine intoxication) is listed first on the final anatomic diagnosis and the laboratory findings that support the diagnosis or certification are listed subsequently. Since laboratory testing usually results in some form of report, the name of the reporting agency and accession number of the laboratory report can be listed as a referent for the readers in case they wish to request a copy of the report for their own edification.

Police reports and further investigation

Interactions with law enforcement are part and parcel to being a death investigator, as has been presented throughout this book, and therefore police reports are an important source of information for casework. Any discussion with law enforcement should not only be documented by the death investigator in writing or in the electronic log, either to be stored in the case file, but also, if any certification decisions are based upon law enforcement findings conveyed by telephonic or personal means, the official police report containing that information should be made part of the case file. This protects the medical examiner/coroner's office from appearing to act outside its purview and acts as a referent for a reader. In fact, there are certain cases where manner of death certification is strictly due to investigative information provided by law enforcement. These are cases where forensic pathologists are not going to talk with the material witnesses as the case is now criminal in nature and, as such, witness interviews are only carried out by law enforcement. In addition, if the investigative information is based on interview with a suspect that was videotaped, the video can and should be viewed by the forensic pathologist prior to certification. If the video is procedurally unable to be viewed, the forensic pathologist should request a copy of the transcript of the interview. In some way, shape, or form the material information gleaned by law enforcement must be documented per-

manently, either electronically or by paper means. Certifying a death as a homicide based on a telephonic conversation can be dangerous and is fraught with potential problems, especially if the detective recants what they discussed telephonically with the forensic pathologist. Thus police reports are very important pieces of investigative information and documentation that should be made freely available to death investigators and forensic pathologists. If law enforcement photographs of the scene, evidence, or official documents and reports are not made available to the forensic pathologist, medical examiner, or coroner and, as such, cause and/or manner determinations cannot be made due to the lack of information, it is appropriate to certify the death as undetermined for the segments in question, as not enough information is available to make a determination within a reasonable degree of medical certainty. When this occurs, the opinion section should reflect the lack of provided information and that if further, probative information is made available the certifier reserves the right to amend the cause and manner of death.

Death certification

When to certify

Certification occurs when the forensic pathologist either has all of the information available regarding the circumstances of a death, *or* has realized that there is no further information to be had or is available to them and has to make a decision based upon their education, experience, training, and the *available* information. There are times when there is no further information that is apparent, and the forensic pathologist is deciding between two manners of death. Some forensic pathologists simply pick the most reasonable one based on their experience and the investigational information available at that time. Other forensic pathologists will simply certify the manner of death as undetermined, with the understanding that upon the receipt of probative information material to the manner of death the manner can be amended to reflect that information.

How to certify

There are at least two different schools of thought on this particular subject. Some forensic pathologists believe that death certification should be as detailed as possible, others believe that only absolutely required facts should be included. In either case, the cause and manner must be *defensible* opinions as they are the basis for insurance payouts, and civil proceedings wherein the cause may be perceived to be a preventable event caused by alleged negligence or work-related phenomena. Thus the cause and manner of death carry the potential for legal proceedings and, as such, must be rendered with an extreme measure of caution and humility. Death certificates (Figure 8.1a through c) have specific parts for demographic and historical information, place of death, time of death, and then the cause and manner of death. Death certificates are generally similar in content as state organizations generally need the same information for Vital Statistics. The format of the certificate varies widely from state to state; however, most have similar sections for the actual death certification and related information.

There is usually a section for the medical certifier (Figure 8.1a) by which the physician indicates whether they are the certifying physician or the medical examiner; a signature section for the physician of record, the date certified, time of death, a medical examiner's case number (when appropriate), the physician's license number, the certifier's name, the name of the attending physician (if different from the certifying physician), the certifier's state, the city or town of certifier's profession, street number of certifier, zip code of certifying physician; signature blocks for the state and county subregistrars, date filed by the subregistrar, the manner of death, indication of whether the medical examiner was contacted due to cause of death, the cause of death (in reverse sequential order to be discussed later), significant "other" conditions that contribute to death, but do not result in the underlying cause of death already given, whether an autopsy was performed, whether autopsy findings were available to complete the cause of death; a section in which to enter surgery if it was included in cause of death or contributing conditions, date of surgery (where appropriate); whether tobacco use contributed to the death; a block, if the decedent is female, to comment on whether there was a pregnancy within the last year; date of injury, time of injury, if the decedent was injured, whether the injury occurred at work, the geographic location of the injury, and if a transportation injury, the position of the decedent and the type of vehicle (see block #30 through 52b on Figure 8.1b).

Focusing on the actual certification part of the death certificate (Box 41, entitled "Cause of Death-Part I" in Figure 8.1c), there is a particular process to addressing the cause of death wherein sequential information is reported with one condition per line, starting with the *most recent* condition on the top line and proceeding chronologically backward on the lines below.

Figure 8.1a Typical death certificate, used with permission of the Bureau of Vital Statistics, Florida.

30. CERTIFIER: **Certifying Physician** - To the best of my knowledge, death occurred at the time, date and place, and due to the cause(s) and manner stated

(Check one)   **Medical Examiner** - On the basis of examination, and/or investigation, in my opinion, death occurred at the time, date and place, and due to the cause(s) and manner stated

31a. *(Signature and Title of Certifier)* ▶	31b. DATE CERTIFIED (Mo., Day, Yr.)	32. TIME OF DEATH (24 hr.)	33. MEDICAL EXAMINER'S CASE NUMBER

34a. LICENSE NUMBER *(of Certifier)*	34b. CERTIFIER'S NAME	35. NAME OF ATTENDING PHYSICIAN *(if other than Certifier)*

36a. CERTIFIER'S - STATE	36b. CITY OR TOWN	36c. STREET AND NUMBER	36d. ZIP CODE

37. SUBREGISTRAR - *Signature and Date* ▶	38a. LOCAL REGISTRAR - *Signature* ▶	38b. DATE FILED BY REGISTRAR (Mo., Day, Yr.)

39. MANNER OF DEATH   The following are under the jurisdiction of the medical examiner   **40. WAS MEDICAL EXAMINER CONTACTED DUE TO CAUSE OF DEATH?** Yes   No

Natural   Accident   Suicide   Homicide   Pending Investigation   Could not be determined

41. CAUSE OF DEATH - PART I (See instructions on back)   Enter the chain of events - diseases, injuries, or complications - that directly caused the death. **DO NOT enter terminal events such as cardiac arrest, respiratory arrest, or ventricular fibrillation without showing the etiology.** DO NOT ABBREVIATE. Enter only one cause on a line.   Approximate Interval: Onset to Death

IMMEDIATE CAUSE (Final disease or condition resulting in death)   a. _____ Due to (or as a consequence of):

Sequentially list conditions, if any, leading to the cause listed on line a. Enter the **UNDERLYING CAUSE LAST** (disease or injury that initiated the events resulting in death)   b. _____ Due to (or as a consequence of):   c. _____ Due to (or as a consequence of):   d. _____

PART II. Enter other significant conditions contributing to death but not resulting in the underlying cause given in PART I.

42a. WAS AN AUTOPSY PERFORMED? Yes ___ No	42b. WERE AUTOPSY FINDINGS AVAILABLE TO COMPLETE THE CAUSE OF DEATH? Yes ___ No

43a. IF SURGERY MENTIONED IN PART I OR II, ENTER REASON FOR SURGERY	43b. DATE OF SURGERY (Mo., Day, Yr.)	44. DID TOBACCO USE CONTRIBUTE TO DEATH? Yes ___ No ___ Probably ___ Unknown

45. IF FEMALE: Not pregnant within past year   Unknown if pregnant within past year   Yes, pregnant within past year *(Select one below):* Pregnant at time of death   Not pregnant at time of death, but pregnant within 42 days of death   Not pregnant at time of death, but pregnant 43 days to 1 year before death

46. DATE OF INJURY (Month, Day, Year)	47. TIME OF INJURY (24 hr.)	48. INJURY AT WORK? Yes ___ No	49a. LOCATION OF INJURY - STATE

49b. CITY OR TOWN	49c. STREET AND NUMBER	49d. APT. NO.	49e. ZIP CODE

50. DESCRIBE HOW INJURY OCCURRED	51. PLACE OF INJURY (e.g. Decedent's home, construction site, restaurant, wooded area)

F TRANSPORTATION INJURY, **52a. Status of Decedent**   Driver/Operator   Passenger   Pedestrian   Other *(Specify)*

52b. Type of Vehicle   Car/Minivan   S.U.V.   Motorcycle   Pickup Truck/Cargo Van   Bus   Heavy Transport   Other *(Specify)*

Figure 8.1b Death certificate sections for certifier, used with permission of the Bureau of Vital Statistics, Florida.

39. MANNER OF DEATH   The following are under the jurisdiction of the medical examiner   **40. WAS MEDICAL EXAMINER CONTACTED DUE TO CAUSE OF DEATH?** Yes   No

Natural   Accident   Suicide   Homicide   Pending Investigation   Could not be determined

41. CAUSE OF DEATH - PART I (See instructions on back)   Enter the chain of events - diseases, injuries, or complications - that directly caused the death. **DO NOT enter terminal events such as cardiac arrest, respiratory arrest, or ventricular fibrillation without showing the etiology.** DO NOT ABBREVIATE. Enter only one cause on a line.   Approximate Interval: Onset to Death

IMMEDIATE CAUSE (Final disease or condition resulting in death)   a. _____ Due to (or as a consequence of):

Sequentially list conditions, if any, leading to the cause listed on line a. Enter the **UNDERLYING CAUSE LAST** (disease or injury that initiated the events resulting in death)   b. _____ Due to (or as a consequence of):   c. _____ Due to (or as a consequence of):   d. _____

PART II. Enter other significant conditions contributing to death but not resulting in the underlying cause given in PART I.

42a. WAS AN AUTOPSY PERFORMED? ___ Yes ___ No	42b. WERE AUTOPSY FINDINGS AVAILABLE TO COMPLETE THE CAUSE OF DEATH? ___ Yes ___ No

Figure 8.1c Cause and manner of death section(s) of death certificate, used with permission of the Bureau of Vital Statistics, Florida.

Thus, the terminal event, or *immediate cause of death* is listed on the top line ((a) in Figure 8.1c); any factor or condition caused by the underlying cause of death and leading to the immediate cause of death, or the *intermediate cause of death* is listed on the middle line(s) ((b) and (c) in Figure 8.1c); the injury, disease, poison, or condition that initiated the chain of events culminating in death, or the *underlying cause of death*, is listed on the bottom line ((d) in Figure 8.1c).

A generic, but illustrative example would be:

Part I

A. Most recent condition
    Due to, or as a consequence of:
B. Next oldest condition
    Due to, or as a consequence of:
C. Oldest (original, initiating) condition.

So, using this logic, a more specific example in an adult would be:

Part I

A. Hemopericardium
    Due to, or as a consequence of:
B. Myocardial infarction with left ventricular rupture
    Due to, or as a consequence of:
C. Arteriosclerotic cardiovascular disease

Thus, in the above example, hemopericardium is the immediate cause of death; myocardial infarction with left ventricular rupture is the intermediate cause of death; and arteriosclerotic cardiovascular disease is the underlying cause of death as it set up the physiologic and anatomic aberrations that culminated in death.

Another example for an infant or child would be:

Part I

A. Pneumonia
    Due to, or as a consequence of:
B. Complications of tetralogy of Fallot

Death certification is an *opinion* based on all available information at the time of certification. That being the case, it is permissible to express uncertainty or use presumption based on the available information, so the use of words such as "probable" or "presumed" is appropriate. Thus an example would be:

Part I

A. Gastrointestinal hemorrhage
    Due to, or as a consequence of:
B. Probable peptic ulcer disease

The real focus should be to determine the correct cause of death, within a reasonable degree of medical certainty, because it determines the manner of death, it results in accurate coding and statistics, it will pass the standards of the local or state Vital Records Department and gives information to families who wish to know more about their loved one's death. Causes of death that are generally unacceptable on their own are "cardiac arrest," "respiratory arrest," "cardiorespiratory arrest," "asystole," "arrhythmia," and "sudden death," *unless* there is a reasonable underlying cause of death that qualifies them (e.g., due to, or as a consequence of, arteriosclerotic cardiovascular disease).

The certifications of infant and child deaths follow the same stream of logic and depart only when the sudden infant death syndrome (SIDS) or sudden unexplained (unexpected) infant death (SUID) is rendered as a cause, in that they carry no meaning and bear no clear or conventionally agreed upon mechanism. In addition, if those non-descript terms are used for certification of the cause of death, what should be utilized as manner of death? Natural? Undetermined? It cannot be natural because if the cause of death is not inherently natural, then the manner cannot be natural and if enough is not known about the cause to determine this, a manner of natural cannot be used to a reasonable degree of medical certainty. Following the same logic, if there is not enough information to come to a clear cause of death in an infant and the certifier wishes to invoke SIDS or SUID and the certifier wishes to use undetermined for manner, why not simply capitulate that a cause of death was not able to be determined to a reasonable degree of medical certainty and certify the death as undetermined for both cause and manner?

Thus if there is no clear cause of death of an infant after complete autopsy, laboratory testing, and scene reconstruction, using "undetermined" as the cause of death is a more appropriate certification. There will be pathologists who argue both sides of this particular issue, but it ultimately comes down to consistent use of logic – and reasonable and defensible terms when certifying deaths.

Upon completion of the investigation and readiness to finalize the case, it is often advisable to contact law enforcement in order to determine if there is any other information that has developed and has been reported to them since your last discussion. In addition, it also permits the forensic pathologist, medical examiner, or coroner to verbally convey their findings and their opinions on the cause and manner of death and to receive some feedback.

It is also this time at which, *in cases where no criminality is suspected*, the forensic pathologist, medical examiner, or coroner should make contact with the parent(s)/caregiver(s)/legally authorized person in order to determine if any probative circumstantial information has been elucidated prior to finalization and, if none has been found, to discuss the final opinion on cause and manner of death. This is also an opportunity given to the parent(s)/caregiver(s)/legally authorized person to ask questions or clarify uncertainties or for the pathologist to discuss genetic issues, anticipatory guidance, or expectant management (if any) as appropriate to the case. In addition, it informs the parent(s)/caregiver(s)/legally authorized person that the death certificate and autopsy report will be signed out soon so they can make the appropriate arrangements with insurance companies and funeral homes.

If *criminality is suspected*, the case information should be likely filtered through the lead detective and the detective can, in turn, be the voice of the investigative information going forward to the family, caregivers, and the media. Some medical examiners and coroners may disagree with this philosophy, but this writer considers it of primary importance to keep the case information in the right hands and to ensure that it is distributed appropriately so as not to perturb the criminal investigation and potential construction of the legal case. In fact, depending on the jurisdiction and the philosophy of the chief medical examiner/coroner, it may be most appropriate to triage inquiry of all types with the statement "All questions should be directed to the XXXX Police Department," which permits law enforcement to devise the statement most appropriate for their criminal case. Again, this is a stylistic issue and there are many appropriate courses of action, but always remember that once information is released, the bell cannot be "unrung," especially in this day of immediate electronic posting and internet availability. Many a news media agency has taken a finalized autopsy report from the hand of the medical examiner or coroner's office administrative assistant and has immediately posted it as a PDF file on their news website. Thus the opinions of the death investigation system are almost immediately under very public scrutiny.

Post-certification processes

Following death certification, signage of the death certificate, and completion of the report, the case is usually filed for future reference. Offices generally have procedures for immediate release of autopsy and associated laboratory reports to all material organizations (i.e., law enforcement, district/state/Commonwealth attorneys, child and family services, etc.). Other interested parties (i.e., families, news media, etc.) usually must request reports in writing and then it is up to the office and prevailing government policy to control access to public records. Some states are public record states and others are not and, as such, the death investigatory office may or may not have the right to release case information to non-material parties. In addition, in some states if the case is considered to be an ongoing investigation, the case information may be exempt from public records requests, despite the state having an open public records policy. This information will have to be reviewed in statute and the state attorney's office is likely the best source of this information. In addition, once this information is known, the public information officer/agent of the death investigatory office as well as the governmental attorney's office (wherein the office is under auspices of the county or state) will have to be notified so that all information channels are clear on the over-riding legal guidance.

Case examples

Case 1

Death report: Three-year-old white male with sudden onset of vomiting and abdominal pain. Family was in car returning home from vacation and made detour to local hospital. Decedent found to be dead on arrival at the Emergency Department.

History: Normal healthy male delivered term. No known substantive medical problems since birth. No suspicion of drugs, foul play, or trauma by investigative findings.

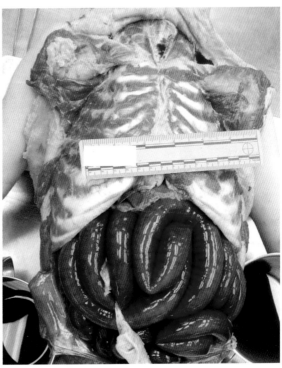

Figure 9.2 Opened peritoneum with dusky, darkened, infarcted small intestine.

Autopsy

Significantly torsed (twisted) mesentery with small intestine infarction. Upon opening, the skin of the trunk demonstrated significant "greening" of the muscle and adipose tissue of the abdomen (Figure 9.1). Further examination of the peritoneal cavity and gastrointestinal tract revealed dusky, darkened infarcted small intestine (Figure 9.2). Further examination revealed a segment of small intestinal mesentery, found to have twisted upon itself (Figure 9.3), obstructing blood flow to the gut. The necrotic small intestinal segments were easily resolved in

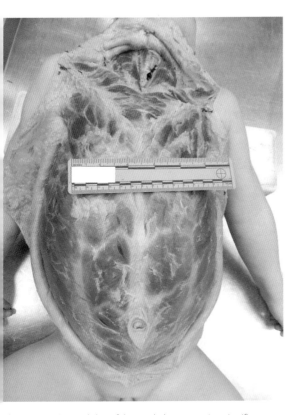

Figure 9.1 Opened skin of the trunk demonstrating significant "greening" of the abdominal soft tissues.

67

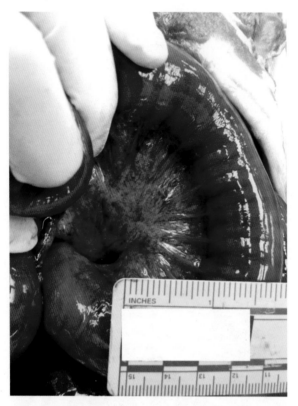

Figure 9.3 Segment of small intestinal mesentery, which was found to be twisted upon itself.

comparison with the grossly normal small intestine (Figure 9.4).

Cause of death: Mesenteric torsion.

Manner of death: Natural.

Discussion

The presentation is sudden and unexpected, reaching two of the cardinal criteria for this to be a death of

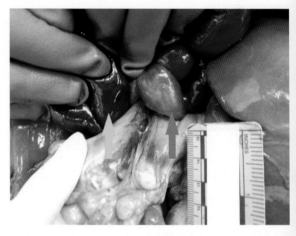

Figure 9.4 Devitalized small intestine (yellow arrow on left side of the photo) next to small intestine which is grossly within normal limits (blue arrow on right side of the photo).

medical examiner/coroner's jurisdiction. The history, as presented here, was completely benign and appears, at least with no other mitigating information, to be natural, but certainly could have been related to some acute intoxication (if the child had recently been given or had surreptitiously ingested medications or illicit drugs), or even a result of accidental or clandestinely inflicted trauma. The best next step following report of this case is to accept jurisdiction and perform radiographs and a full autopsy and be prepared for any eventuality.

Autopsy ruled out trauma in this case in which sudden onset abdominal symptoms in child could suggest etiologies spanning from natural to traumatic, which may or may not be readily appreciated from external exam.

Case 2

Death report: Six- to nine-month-old skeletonized infant found in wooden box (Figure 9.5) under porch of a home.

History: The parents in this case were under investigation for alleged neglect of other living children. The police performed a search of the home looking for evidence of maltreatment and found a box containing the remains of a small child. The home was judged to be in unsanitary and deplorable conditions, and the living children were found to have been kept in cages.

Autopsy

X-rays of the box were taken. A thorough layer-by-layer dissection and documentation of the contents of the box was performed. A small amount of adipocere, bug casings, and strands of fine hair were collected for possible toxicology analysis. The skeleton was laid out and a forensic anthropologist was requested for consultation. The purpose of the anthropology consultation was to determine:

1. Age/gender
2. Completeness of skeleton
3. Evidence of pathology (natural or traumatic)
4. Recovery of bone for DNA for possible paternity/maternity issues
5. The time period the child had been dead and in the box

The autopsy findings in conjunction with the anthropological consultation were:

1. Skeletonized infant with no residual tissue
2. Toxicology on microscopic pieces of oxidized fat, hair, and adjacent insects and casings were found to be non-contributory

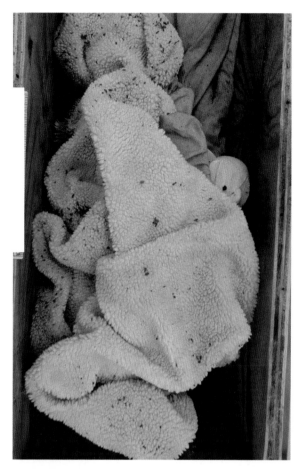

Figure 9.6 Personal items discovered inside the box as it was opened.

3. No skeletal trauma
4. Skeletal findings suggestive of iron deficiency anemia

Cause of death: Undetermined.

Manner of death: Undetermined.

Discussion

Evaluation of the wooden box and its contents (Figures 9.6 and 9.7) demonstrated the skeletal remains of a six- to nine-month-old infant, which was dressed and diapered (Figure 9.8), wrapped in a blanket, and placed within the box with a stuffed animal. This arrangement suggests some level of care by whomever placed the infant in the box, but was by no means indicative of it. Examination of the skeleton demonstrated no stigmata of perimortem trauma, but

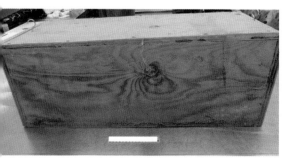

Figure 9.5 Box found under the porch of a home.

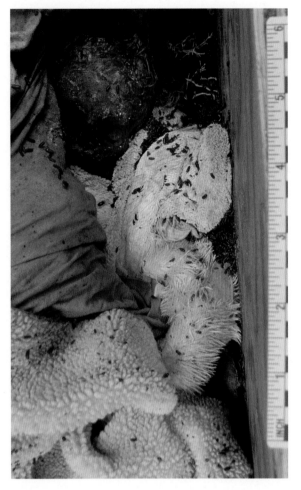

Figure 9.7 Skull discovered upon examination of contents of the box.

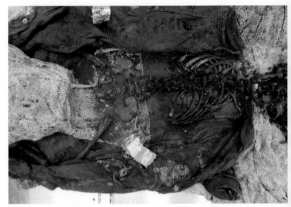

Figure 9.8 Skeletal remains of an infant with a diaper on and dressed appropriately.

suggested to the forensic anthropologist indications of iron deficiency anemia. In light of the deplorable conditions of the home and the state of abuse/neglect of the living children, the context of this death may very well have been homicidal in nature. However, with no other indications either investigationally (e.g., admissions of beating or suffocating the child) or anatomically (e.g., indicia of antemortem fractures), this death

was certified undetermined for both cause and manner. Depending on the context in which skeletonized remains are found, the cause of these deaths could also be appropriately certified as "violence of undetermined origin" and the manner certified as homicide. The aforementioned cause of death is generally reserved for those deaths in which skeletonized remains are found in a place or situation that suggests to the certifier a degree of suspicion for volitionally inflicted injury or neglect and the concealment of the body to hide these actions. These certifications are rare (in the experience of the authors), but are useful to describe certain situations where autopsy of the remains demonstrates no anatomic cause of death, but wherein the body is discovered in a context worrisome for homicidal violence. In cases involving skeletal remains it is best to consult with an experienced anthropologist. The forensic anthropologist provided vital investigatory information, such as age range estimation and gender, and was able to assist the medical examiner to assess the remains for trauma. Forensic pathology often requires a multidisciplinary approach. The use of additional experts can be extremely valuable to the investigation of a death.

Case 3

Death report: Normally developed, previously healthy one-year-old black toddler with reported sudden onset of vomiting and flu-like symptoms.

History: The decedent's uncle, who was reportedly babysitting the infant, reported that the child became acutely ill (i.e., vomiting, abdominal pain) prior to becoming acutely unresponsive. The child was taken to the Emergency Department via Fire Rescue and was found to be dead on arrival. The clinical working diagnosis, given the history they had recorded, was viral infection – due to no external findings of anything to the contrary and no reported history of trauma, abuse, foul play, or any suspicion of drug intoxication.

Autopsy

1. Protruding, red-appearing anus
2. Thymic hemorrhage
3. Posterior liver laceration

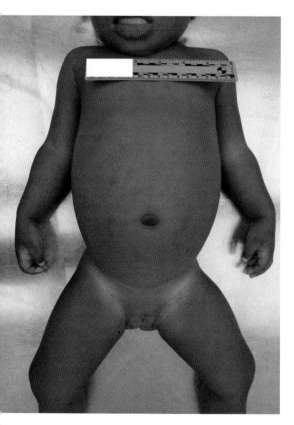

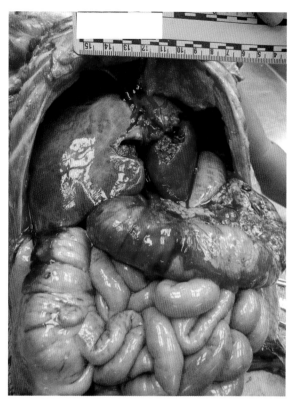

Figure 9.10 Abdominal viscera with marked soft tissue hemorrhage and indication of liver laceration.

4. Pancreatic contusion
5. Hemoperitoneum (600 mL)
6. Multiple posterior rib fractures

Cause of death: Blunt force injury of abdomen.

Manner of death: Homicide.

Discussion

Due to the protruding anus a sexual assault kit was collected. Given the clinical suspicion of infection, culture specimens were collected from the airway. The abdomen was distended and the abdominal skin demonstrated scattered contusions (Figure 9.9). A layerwise abdominal/chest dissection demonstrated no hemorrhage. Opening the abdomen revealed blood collected within the peritoneal cavity (hemoperitoneum) and visceral soft tissue hemorrhage (Figure 9.10) due to lacerations of the liver (Figure 9.11) and contusion of the pancreas (Figure 9.12). The police were notified during the

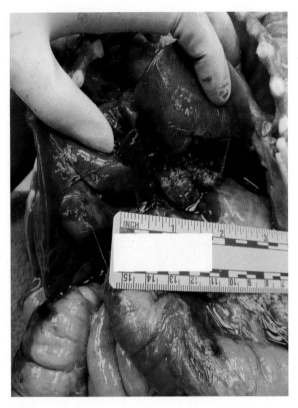

Figure 9.11 Posterior aspect of the liver with capsular and parenchymal laceration and soft tissue hemorrhage.

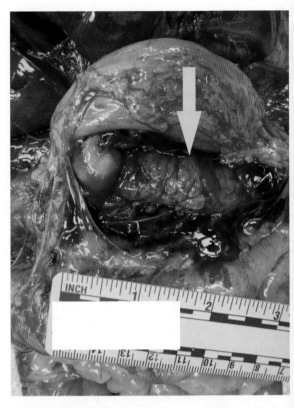

Figure 9.12 Pancreas (yellow arrow) surrounded by marked soft tissue hemorrhage.

autopsy regarding the suspicion of trauma to the child. The police questioned whether the injuries could be due to resuscitation artifact. It was explained that the lacerations are extensive, and the pancreas is deep to contuse by resuscitation, and are unlikely the result of chest compressions in the Emergency Department.

In this particular case, the investigatory information and medical history were incongruent with the anatomic findings of blunt force injuries of the abdomen. Following the autopsy, the decedent's uncle subsequently admitted to one "kick" to the abdomen, which reportedly caused the child to travel "several feet" and to strike a fixed object within the room.

Thereafter the decedent reportedly would not stop crying.

Blood cultures were collected despite the presence of the physical injuries in order to rule out a possible coinciding infection and for completeness. The results were negative for infection.

In this case the clinical suspicion was the child had succumbed to an infectious process. The autopsy demonstrated clear signs of trauma. At times a seemingly routine autopsy of a sick child can become a homicide investigation. The absence of external injuries should not rule out the possibility of inflicted trauma in the mind of the pathologist.

Case 4

Death report: Ten-day-old white male who was the product of an uncomplicated pregnancy and delivery despite a mother with a history of addiction.

History: The infant was reportedly found unresponsive, positioned upright in a car seat at home. The decedent's mother (caretaker) was a poor historian with a history of acute substance abuse.

Autopsy

1. Acute bronchopneumonia
2. Postmortem nasal viral cultures positive for parainfluenza virus
3. Large intestinal situs inversus (incidental)
4. No anatomic evidence of lethal trauma

Cause of death: Complications of parainfluenza

Manner of death: Natural

Discussion

Autopsy permitted death investigators to anatomically and toxicologically evaluate the decedent in order to determine a cause of death and to give benchmarks with which to correlate historic information with external findings (i.e., positioning). In this case, despite the paucity of information available from the caretaker(s), the reportedly benign investigational information was in agreement with the lack of demonstrable trauma anatomically. In addition, performance of the autopsy permitted microbiological testing to be performed and to be correlated with histologic findings. This logical and methodical approach permitted the elucidation of a viral infection that caused acute bronchopneumonia, which, in turn, caused the death of this infant. One can see that without the anatomic examination and proper laboratory testing, no cause of death would have been able to be certified in this case. In addition, one can already see that there is a wide range of clinical histories and investigational information that is gathered in each case, but that proper certification requires anatomic evaluation in order to correlate all the relevant information and to propose reasonably logical and meaningful causes and manners of death.

Case 5

Death report: Toddler with bruises on arrival at house of family friend who suddenly became unresponsive.

History: The decedent was a 15-month-old Caucasian female toddler who lived with her mother but, on occasion, she was left in the custody of a male friend and his family while the mother would take time for personal affairs. On a Friday evening in December, this toddler was left with the friend and his family for several days. Upon arrival at the friend's home, the toddler was noticed to have many bruises on various areas of her body. There was no discernible or described pattern to the bruising, and over the next four days there were periods where she was reportedly witnessed to stumble and fall, hitting her head on several occasions. On the fifth day, while being bathed by her caregiver, the toddler had a sudden loss of consciousness and paramedics were called to resuscitate the toddler. When the Emergency Medical Services responders arrived, the toddler was found to be unresponsive without pulse or respiration. Aggressive attempts at resuscitation by both the paramedics and the hospital personnel were unsuccessful and she was pronounced dead shortly after admission to the Emergency Department. No blood or urine samples were collected in the hospital prior to the toddler's death.

Autopsy

Medical examiner autopsy report

A. Blunt force head trauma:

1. bilateral subdural hematomas
2. diffuse subarachnoid hemorrhage
3. cerebral edema and contusions
4. marked optic nerve sheath hemorrhage
5. focal retinal hemorrhages, bilateral
6. large right-sided cephalohematoma
7. focal left-sided subgaleal contusions
8. multiple contusions and focal abrasion of the head, face, ears, lips, mouth, and neck.

B. Multiple fresh and older contusions of the trunk and extremities.

C. Focal circular pattern of thermal injury on the dorsum of the left foot.

Medical examiner reported

Cause of death: Non-accidental blunt force head trauma.

Manner of death: Homicide.

Private forensic analysis added

A. A contusion on the right forehead attributed to a trip and fall in the living area of the caregiver's home on day two of the visit (witnessed by the family).

B. A recent elliptically shaped abrasion with associated contusion in the parietal region (top of head) just to the left of the midline and a contusion anterior (toward forehead) on both the right and left sides of the midline. This group of injuries is attributed a fall in the backyard on day three when the toddler was first knocked backward by the family dog and then got up and fell forward onto a weight set (witnessed by family).

C. An edematous subscalpular and subgaleal hematoma located on the right posterior temporal and parietal regions (above and behind the right ear) was due to impact on a metal bed rail. This injury is attributed to a witnessed fall on day three subsequent to the fall described in above in paragraph "B." This fall occurred when the caregiver's son was pulling himself up on the toddler causing her to fall backward hitting her head on a metal bed rail.

D. Parallel, diagonally oriented contusions involving the left lateral orbital facial skin with extension onto the left lateral forehead and superior helix of the left ear. This injury is attributed to the toddler falling from the bed on day four of the visit. She had been napping and was found on the floor next to the bed.

E. There was no evidence of sexual assault.

F. There was a small frenulum tear, excoriation and abrasions, and contusions of the lips and inner aspect of the mouth. These were all attributed to intubation and the resuscitative efforts and/or the fall out of the bed.

G. Internal examination of the head disclosed no evidence of skull fracture, but there were bilateral subdural hematomas greater on the right than the left (70 cc total) composed of both clotted and non-clotted blood. There was diffuse subarachnoid hemorrhage most prominent over the cerebral convexities, cerebral edema, and multiple irregular cortical contusions on the right and left inferior temporal lobes. Subarachnoid hemorrhage was seen on the brain stem and cerebellum. When the brain was sectioned following fixation, no deep white matter hemorrhages were found.

H. Microscopic assessment of the subdural hematoma showed autolyzed blood consistent with a subacute hematoma suggesting the subdural hemorrhage occurred more than 48 hours prior to death. The iron stain of the subdural hematoma was focally positive. These findings correlated with the microscopic dating of the brain injury.

I. Microscopic assessment:

1. Cerebral cortical and cerebellar sections disclosed subarachnoid hemorrhage infiltrated by neutrophils and macrophages with the iron stain showing scattered macrophages with intracytoplasmic iron granules.

2. Cerebral cortical sections showed scattered subpial intraparenchymal hemorrhages, and in the adjacent non-hemorrhagic parenchyma there were scattered, isolated, neutrophils and occasional perivascular mononuclear cell infiltrates.

3. In the neocortex, the neuronal architecture was normal while examination of the areas of underlying hemorrhage showed shrunken and hyperchromatic neurons. The iron stain was negative. The immunohistochemical stain CD-68 confirmed the infiltration by macrophages and neutrophils. The factor VIII stain was not contributory.

4. The eye sections showed small petechial hemorrhages involving the optic nerve, the retinal ganglion cell layer, and the outer nuclear layer. One of two eye sections showed more hemorrhage with separation of the retinal ganglion cell layer from the deeper layers along the outer plexiform layer. The iron stain was positive only for this latter eye, but there were aggregates of CD-68-positive mononuclear cells in both eyes and optic nerves.

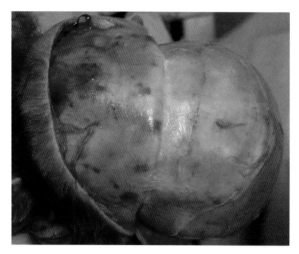

Figure 9.13 Contusions of the reflected fontal scalp.

J. No blood was drawn from the toddler in the Emergency Department and postmortem coagulation studies could not be performed. The diffuse bruising pattern consisted of round to oval superficial contusions. Except for the right posterior temporal and parietal subscalpular/subgaleal hematoma found above and behind the right ear, there were no patterned or deep contusions as often seen in intentionally inflicted trauma.

Consultative cause and manner of death

Cause of death: Blunt force head and brain trauma complicated by consumptive disseminated intravascular coagulopathy, hypovolemic shock, and multiorgan system failure.

Manner of death: Undetermined versus accident.

Discussion

The distribution of the contusions and abrasions found on the toddler was not thought to represent an inflicted abusive blunt trauma pattern, but rather, a distribution of "bruises" expected and seen in patients with consumptive disseminated intravascular coagulopathy or "DIC." Analysis of the autopsy photographs disclosed numerous clusters of random contusions (Figures 9.13 and 9.14) with no clear patterned injuries, consistent with inflicted trauma, such as from a blunt object, e.g., a belt, coat hanger, whip, club, or similar object. In addition, the child was found to have bilateral

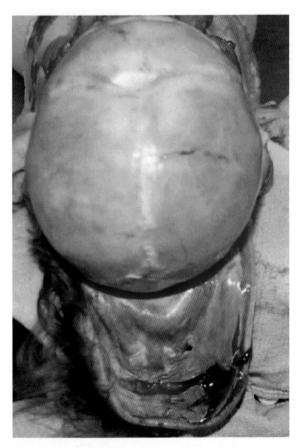

Figure 9.14 Contusion of the reflected occipital scalp.

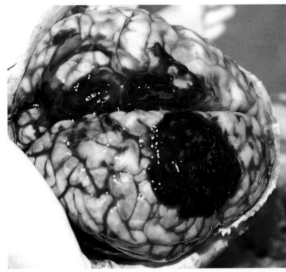

Figure 9.15 Surface of the cerebral cortex with bilateral subdural hematomata.

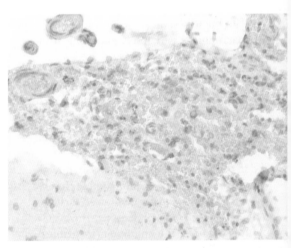

Figure 9.16 Section of cerebral cortex stained with anti-CD-68 antibodies highlighting the macrophages (brown cytoplasmic staining) admixed within the inflammatory infiltrate.

subdural hematomata (Figure 9.15). The skeletal X-ray survey was negative with no recent, healing, or healed fractures as sometimes seen in child abuse victims. In addition, sections of cerebral cortex stained with anti-CD-68 antibodies (specific for macrophages) demonstrated positivity in the inflammatory infiltrate, indicating that the hematomatas were not acute (Figure 9.16).

The paramedics testified they did not see any injuries on the toddler at the caregiver's residence when they responded to the emergency call. Careful examination of all contusions disclosed patterns consistent with therapeutic resuscitative efforts, corroborating the paramedic's observations.

The historical background in this case was examined and all injuries were correlated with the reported accidental injuries while in the care and custody of the male caregiver and his family. This case was thoroughly examined by a Board-certified forensic pathologist and a Board-certified neuropathologist with extensive forensic experience.

The "stress response to trauma," is the body's reaction to injury where there is activation of hormonal and metabolic systems following injury or trauma (Desborough, 2000). The response to tissue and vascular injury includes activation of (1) the coagulation system to seal injured blood vessels and prevent excessive blood loss and (2) the inflammatory/immunologic system to initiate repair and defense against infection. At time of injury tissue thromboplastin (TTP) initiates the coagulation cascade at the site of injury by converting prothrombin to thrombin in the presence of Ca^{2+}, resulting in blood clot formation. Coagulation disorders including DIC are well known complications of head injury (HI) and the rich source of TTP in brain tissue may be responsible for onset of post-HI coagulopathy and delayed brain changes, such as cerebral contusion and hematomata (Pathak *et al.*, 2005). With the onset of DIC, there is a pathologic consumption of the blood clotting proteins due to the futile cycle of clot formation and clot lysis. If this consumptive coagulopathy is not recognized and treated in concert with treatment of the inciting traumatic head injury, the patient may develop hypovolemic shock and multiorgan system failure resulting in death.

In this case, the toddler was thought to have multiple injuries to her head and brain over a three- to six-day period with no severe acute trauma occurring in the 24- to 48-hour period prior to death. The postmortem diagnosis of consumptive DIC was made by correlating the physical findings and the toddler's rapid clinical deterioration without response to resuscitation. Other than the blunt head trauma, there was no underlying organ or systemic pathology that was determined to cause this toddler's death.

Outcome

The male caregiver was charged with first degree murder and bound over for trial. At trial, the caregiver was found not guilty of all charges and acquitted.

Comment by authors

Careful anatomic and historic evaluation of all head trauma in infants and toddlers is required to avoid improper classification of the manner of death. It is important to collect as much antecedent information as is possible in these cases. Collection of *all* medical records (as the decedent was only 15 months old), a careful history of the decedent's behaviors, routines, and any trauma prior to the period of potential lethal injury and *independent* accounts of witnesses (if they exist) during the time between last known period of baseline health and behavior to the period when the decedent began manifesting symptoms, are the first, best approaches to take in these cases. The goal should be to account for the decedent as much as is possible during the time period before death in order to determine the presence of any antecedent events that may explain any injuries found. In addition, neuropathology consultation and documentation photography are advisable in cases where a clear injury pattern is not easily discerned or in cases where there is difficulty resolving whether anatomic findings are injurious, natural, or artifactual. In addition, in order to better resolve the etiology of difficult-to-categorize anatomic findings, they must be correlated with the antecedent history in order to build a context for those findings. Because of the differences in the training and experiences of each death investigator, there can be differences in the "weights" given to the veracity of historic information related to injuries documented at autopsy. In this particular case, one should be concerned at the sheer number of head injuries the aforementioned decedent was reported to have suffered in a relatively short span of time and that the *number* of these head injuries in that timespan (rather than their aggregate severity or their potential anatomic or physiologic magnitude) may indicate a more suspicious context and may argue for a more thorough investigation of the circumstances. There are often surrogate markers for suspicious or "criminally injurious" activities within these cases, and if the death investigator's experience is such that their curiosity is triggered by a lack of reasonable explanation for documented injuries, law enforcement and other elements of the criminal justice system should be alerted and the investigation should be maintained until the circumstances are resolved. If the circumstances are not resolved to the satisfaction of the death investigator, the cause and manner of death certification of undetermined is a reasonable and logical conclusion.

Case 6

Death report: The decedent was a 6½-month-old infant with blunt force head trauma.

History: The decedent was a 6½-month-old infant male who lived with his biological mother and father and two-year-old brother in a garage converted into an apartment. The floor was concrete and was covered by a thin carpet. On the day of the incident, the two minor children were in the care and custody of their father while the children's mother was at work. During the early evening hours the decedent sustained severe blunt force head injury when, according to the father, the 6½-month-old was accidently dropped – falling an estimated 4 feet onto the carpet-covered concrete floor.

Shortly after the impact, the infant became unresponsive and emergency medical services were called. When Emergency Medical Services arrived at the scene, the infant was apneic and bradycardiac and within two minutes went into pulseless electrical activity. The infant was successfully resuscitated and then transported to a children's hospital for diagnosis and treatment. On admission, the infant was unresponsive with a Glasgow Coma Scale score of 3; his pupils were fixed, dilated, and unequal; his mean arterial blood pressure was in the low 40s; he was apneic; and he had marked acidemia.

The diagnostic CT scan showed a left occipital scalp hematoma, a non-displaced right occipital bone fracture, and mild widening of the left lambdoid suture versus non-displaced fracture. There was (1) extensive acute subdural hemorrhage along the vertex measuring in thickness 10 mm on the right and 6 mm on the left; (2) a small subacute hematoma in the right cerebral convexity 4 mm thick; (3) mild subarachnoid hemorrhage on the right vertex, right temporal region, and posterior aspect of the interhemispheric fissure; and (4) mild cerebral edema with minimal ventricular effacement without midline shift or herniation. The CT scan of the cervical spine showed no evidence of fracture or subluxation. The skeletal survey was otherwise negative for fractures or other pathology.

The infant was admitted in critical condition and his hospital course was one of rapid deterioration. The eye examination disclosed bilateral retinal hemorrhages without retinoschisis, and the decedent subsequently developed a coagulopathy with an elevated PT, aPTT, INR, low fibrinogen, and low normal platelet counts. The follow-up CT scan disclosed marked increase in the subdural hematoma with new acute subdural hematoma along the tentorium, increased diffuse cerebral edema with findings of diffuse anoxic injury and effacement of the lateral ventricles. Despite aggressive management, the infant died on the second hospital day.

During the incident investigation, the father gave the sheriff's detectives different accounts of how his infant son fell. The father initially said he was in the kitchen holding the infant in one arm and his two-year-old in his other arm. By his report, the older boy began to squirm pushing against the father causing the father to lose his balance and to drop the infant who fell to the floor and rapidly lost consciousness.

When the detectives told the father that the infant's injuries could not be caused by a fall, the father then said he was holding the older son in one arm and his younger son was in his car seat. When he tried to pick him up out of the seat, he said the infant slipped and fell out of the car seat, causing his head to bounce back and forth on the floor.

The detectives then told the father his second explanation did not match his son's injuries and suggested to the father that he "shook" his son. The father then lowered his head and whispered he was afraid to say what happened because he was afraid of getting in trouble. The father said he had indeed shaken his son because he was a fussy baby crying all the time, and this frustrated the father because he could not make him stop crying. The father said he shook his young son, but not for very long, and his son fell out of his arms, falling onto the ground, hitting his head on the concrete floor covered by a thin carpet.

Autopsy

A. Head trauma:

1. bilateral semi-circular occipital skull fractures, inferior to the lambdoid sutures
2. diffuse occipital subcutaneous/galeal hemorrhage
3. occipital periosteal hemorrhage is geographic and diffuse, more prominent on left
4. bilateral subdural hemorrhage, 20 cc total, left side greater
5. right and left eyes: mild intra-retinal hemorrhage, left eye, iron stain negative
6. neuropathologic diagnoses:

a. suggestive evidence of blunt force traumatic injury to head

b. residual right greater than left huge subdural parafalcine hemorrhage

c. bilateral subarachnoid hemorrhage, acute in convexity extending through interhemispheric fissure

d. generalized cerebral edema, mild to moderate

B. Skin findings:

1. light purple contusion over right mandible
2. light purple contusion over left mandible
3. very faint blue contusion superior to the left brow
4. dark purple contusion of upper mid forehead
5. hypo-pigmented area over thyroid cartilage, possibly scar, negative for subcutaneous hemorrhage
6. purple discoloration over the right buttock. Autopsy incision negative for subcutaneous hemorrhage

C. Radiology consult:

1. bilateral occipital bone fracture, no radiographic healing changes
2. remaining skeletal structures normal and negative for radiographic evidence of abusive or inflicted trauma
3. no evidence of significant congenital or developmental skeletal anomaly

Medical examiner reported

Cause of death: Blunt head trauma.

Manner of death: Homicide.

Private forensic analysis

A. Blunt force head trauma to occiput manifested by:

1. occipital subcutaneous and subgaleal acute hemorrhage, greater on left than right
2. recent (acute), bilateral, semi-circular occipital bone fractures, greater on left than right
3. occipital periosteal acute hemorrhage, diffuse, greater on left than right
4. subdural hemorrhage, acute parafalcine, 20 cc total, left greater than right

5. subarachnoid hemorrhage, acute bilateral in convexity extending through interhemispheric fissure
6. mild to moderate cerebral edema
7. right and left eyes: mild intra-retinal hemorrhage, left eye, iron stain negative
8. abnormal coagulation studies, consistent with onset of disseminated intravascular coagulopathy (DIC)

B. Skin:

1. faint contusions, consistent with medical intervention and resuscitative efforts
2. no evidence of inflicted trauma

C. Skeletal survey:

1. negative for fractures, except for acute skull fracture
2. no radiographic evidence of neck injury

Consultative cause and manner of death

Cause of death: Blunt force head trauma complicated by acute subdural hemorrhage and cerebral edema.

Manner of death: Accident.

Discussion

This case highlights a number of controversial points regarding accidental and inflicted pediatric head injury. It was the opinion of the consulting forensic pathologist that this case was not "shaken baby syndrome (SBS)." This opinion was based on several factors, one being the absence of neck injury found radiographically or at autopsy, and in the absence of neck injury, SBS can be excluded, according to some sources (Duhaime *et al.*, 1987; Prange *et al.*, 2003). This opinion is often debated as other sources claim that injury to the cervical spinal cord can occur in 15 to 20% of shaking cases (Orner, personal communication). A recent paper suggests that cervical nerve root hemorrhages occur in 100% of shaking cases (Matshes *et al.*, 2011). This paper includes twelve cases of hyperextension/hyperflexion injury in children. Of the twelve cases, five were "suspected abuse" and two were "admitted abuse." Nine of the twelve children had survival intervals from many hours to several days. The control group is comprised of 23 children with no history of blunt injury. Three of the 23 children survived from three days to twelve days. One of the three children (seven-day survival) had a cervical nerve root injury. It is possible that the high incidence of cervical nerve root injuries seen in this cohort is the result of herniation injury due to cerebral edema as many of the cases experienced lengthy survival intervals. Due to the discrepancy between the published studies, care should be taken when interpreting cervical nerve root hemorrhages.

The differential diagnosis in this case includes "inflicted" blunt force head injury versus blunt force head injury due to accidental fall. If the decedent was subjected to shaking of any degree, it was likely minor due to the absence of neck injury.

When parents admit to "shaking" their infant, this suggests a violent, temper-driven action, when, in fact, the parent might be shaking the infant or toddler trying to illicit an arousal response. Such events should not be taken as a sentinel sign of abuse, and such statements must be analyzed in context of the case findings, to avoid misinterpretation and an erroneous conclusion. Intentional, "non-accidental" severe shaking often causes neck injury (Matshes *et al.*, 2011) and, in this case, neck injury was not appreciated. There is an impact site and skull fracture correlating with the clinical history.

There was a paucity of external injury, and the faint contusions as noted by the medical examiner were felt by the consulting pathologist to be consistent with medical manipulation and resuscitative efforts. There is clinical evidence the decedent had onset of disseminated intravascular coagulopathy (DIC) due to his head injury, and this clotting disorder will have a tendency to augment light bruising from any contact from therapeutic manipulation or during resuscitative efforts. There are (1) no deep contusions; (2) no injuries in varying stages of healing or resolution; and (3) no fractures other than the acute skull fracture.

The retinal hemorrhages were thought to be due to an increase in intracranial pressure. If these hemorrhages were due to trauma, the opinion of the consulting pathologist is that the trauma would have been severe and evident. Retinal and/or optic nerve sheath hemorrhages do not independently indicate an infant or child was abused. In the absence of compelling external trauma, their presence only indicates there was an increase in intracranial pressure.

Correlating the investigative, hospital, and autopsy information supports the clinical history of an

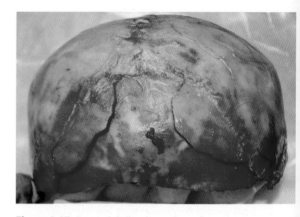

Figure 9.17 Occipital skull with curvilinear fractures.

accidental drop from a height. Although not common, short falls can cause severe injuries.

In this case, the decedent had an impact site to his occiput just left of the midline, and there is no external evidence of injury, i.e., contusion or laceration of the skin. There is a "bump" described on the back of the decedent's head due to the impact and the resultant subgaleal hematoma. Directly beneath this impact site are two curvilinear fractures of the occipital bone (Figure 9.17). The fractures are not depressed as may be expected if the decedent had been struck by a blunt force instrument or struck against the wall or floor.

The independent neuropathologic examination and reconstruction of the decedent's injuries was somewhat impeded because of the following: (1) no gross description of the decedent's internal head injury by the examining medical examiner; (2) no gross photographs of the decedent's brain once the calvarium was removed; (3) no gross photographs of the decedent's brain in the fresh state after removal; (4) no gross photographs of the interior of the decedent's skull; and (5) no gross photographs of the fixed brain either before or during brain cutting. Although there are no standards for the number of microscopic sections to be examined, only four microscopic sections for neuropathologic examination were examined when most examiners will examine seven to ten microscopic slides. However, the examining neuropathologist made the following diagnoses:

1. suggestive evidence of blunt force traumatic injury to head
2. residual right greater than left huge subdural parafalcine hemorrhage

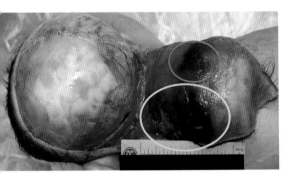

Figure 9.18 Occipital skull with overlying scalp contusions (circled).

3. bilateral subarachnoid hemorrhage, acute, and convexity extending through interhemispheric fissure

4. generalized cerebral edema, mild to moderate.

The infant's scalp impact is depicted in Figure 9.18. The impact site is to the left of the midline causing the larger subgaleal hemorrhage (Figure 9.18, yellow circle). The impact force causes a slightly depressed curvilinear left occipital bone skull fracture with transmission of the impact force through the skull and into the intracranial contents, i.e. the dura mater and brain. The brain cannot compress to absorb the impact force, and the energy must be distributed and transferred in a rebound fashion causing a mirror burst or outward curvilinear skull fracture in the opposite right side of the occipital bone. The fracture impacts the galea resulting in the smaller subgaleal contusion (Figure 9.18, green circle).

There is an absence of autopsy information making reconstruction and evaluation of the traumatic findings difficult. This, in concert with the neuropathologist's opinion, which is that the injuries are "suggestive evidence of blunt force traumatic injury to head," does not suggest homicide as the manner of death. There is, in fact, no doubt that the injuries are due to blunt force injuries. The investigatory data presented and known at the time of the case certification does not suggest to the consulting pathologist that the decedent's death was due to an intentional act, but rather an accidental one.

Consultant conclusion and opinion

1. Cause of death: blunt force head trauma complicated by acute subdural hemorrhage and cerebral edema.
2. The manner of death: accident.
3. The medical evidence supports the history of fall.
4. There is no persuasive evidence the decedent had been physically mishandled or abused.

Comment by authors

Correlation of the injuries with the history or investigative information is mandatory to avoid misinterpretation or overinterpretation of the injuries. Witnesses and potential defendants *may* change their historical observation when interviewed by law enforcement for benign reasons such as fear or feeling responsible (or being made to feel responsible) for an accidental injury. Witnesses and defendants may also change their stories in order to fit them into what they think law enforcement or the death investigators want to hear in order to minimize the perceived magnitude of the injuries they, themselves, have caused. The autopsy findings were not felt to support "shaken baby syndrome" or "shaken impact syndrome" as the mechanism of injury – the mechanism was simply blunt injury to the head. With the anatomic findings and levels of police investigation present in this case, the manner of death may also be certified as "undetermined" due to lack of investigatory information suggestive of homicidal violence in the face of injuries, the source(s) of which are rather unclear and attributable to accidental and non-accidental means. In the authors' experience, when the suspect begins to change their story to fit what they believe law enforcement wants to hear, the veracity of any story they tell must be questioned and the case should be investigated as stringently as is possible in order to elucidate surreptitious abusive injuries. The thought must remain in one's mind that in truly benign circumstances, any reasonable person would give the entire truth at the initial interview, though this does not always happen, despite the reasonability of the caregiver(s).

Case 7

Death report: Nine-week-old infant who became unresponsive.

History: The decedent was a 9-week 3-day-old infant female who had an uneventful spontaneous vaginal delivery to a 17-year-old, primigravida woman. She was reported to be growing and developing normally when, in early November, she began grunting in the morning, her head was reportedly "falling down," and she was vomiting. Three days after onset of symptoms, she was seen by her pediatrician, because she was acting fussy, vomiting, having spells of "not breathing," and she had right leg pain. The parents denied history of sleep habit changes, recent trauma, shaking, falls, or seizures. The doctor's examination was negative with no decreased activity, trauma, or acute distress. He diagnosed neonatal feeding problems due to formula intolerance. The doctor recommended a formula change and the parents complied.

Two days after her doctor's visit, the decedent was found "unresponsive" by her father. She was taken to a nearby medical center with complaints of constitutional fever, vomiting, and decreased activity, and she was described as limp and listless. The admitting diagnosis was sepsis probably due to meningitis. A lumbar puncture was attempted, but failed, and this procedure was never revisited. Her admission laboratory data showed metabolic acidosis, anemia, hyponatremia, elevated white blood cell count with left shift, and elevated blood glucose. On physical examination, the decedent responded to painful stimuli by crying, and then became very lethargic with flaccid upper extremities.

Once stabilized, the decedent was transferred to a children's hospital where she remained unconscious, responding to painful stimuli with a shrill cry. She was severely hypotonic and "floppy" with dilated sluggish pupils, and ophthalmologic examination disclosed severe, bilateral retinal hemorrhage with retinal detachment. The imaging studies showed extensive subarachnoid hemorrhage and subdural hemorrhage, diffuse cerebral edema, and left temporal lobe intraparenchymal hemorrhage. The infant bone survey disclosed no evidence of fractures or other significant abnormality. The infectious disease consultation opined there was no evidence of infection. The decedent was maintained on mechanical ventilation and supportive care, but her condition continued to deteriorate, and she was pronounced dead.

Autopsy

A. Blunt force trauma, head and neck:

1. faint contusions of bilateral upper neck
2. diffuse subdural hemorrhage
3. diffuse subarachnoid hemorrhage:

   a. cerebral convexities
   b. cerebellar hemispheres
   c. brain stem
   d. spinal cord

4. epidural hemorrhage of superior cervical spinal cord
5. diffuse traumatic axonal injury, manifested by β-APP(+) axonal swellings:

   a. posterior limb of internal capsule; bilateral
   b. periventricular white matter; scattered
   c. medulla

6. bilateral tonsillar herniation
7. global hypoxic/ischemic encephalopathy
8. blunt force trauma, eyes

   a. bilateral optic nerve sheath hemorrhages
   b. bilateral retinal hemorrhages

9. macular retinal folds
10. blunt trauma, thorax and abdomen
11. multiple healing rib fractures
12. subdural and epidural hemorrhage of thoracic and lumbar spinal cord

Medical examiner reported

Cause of death: Complications of blunt force head injury.

Manner of death: Homicide.

Private forensic analysis

A. Brain:

1. acute meningitis; evolving or under treatment
2. cerebral edema; marked
3. thrombosis of superior sagittal sinus
4. hemorrhage in lateral ventricles; bilaterally and third ventricle
5. intraparenchymal hemorrhage into bilateral basal ganglia, frontal and occipital lobes with associated softening

6. intermittent, thin layer subdural hemorrhage, cerebral hemispheres; bilateral
7. subarachnoid hemorrhage:
   a. cerebral hemispheres; focal
   b. cerebellar hemispheres; focal
   c. brain stem
8. global hypoxic/ischemic encephalopathy
9. multiple foci of axonal injury; manifest by β-APP(+) swellings:
   a. posterior limb of internal capsule; bilateral
   b. periventricular white matter; scattered
   c. medulla

B. Spinal cord:
   1. focal epidural hemorrhage, upper thoracic, lumbar, and cauda equina (by autopsy photographs)
   2. subdural hemorrhage, described as entire length of spinal cord (no photograph)

C. Skin discoloration on autopsy photographs (not incised or examined microscopically):
   1. oval faint purple–green on right upper neck just beneath mandible
   2. oval very faint purple–green on left upper neck just beneath mandible

D. Eyes:
   1. bilateral optic nerve sheath hemorrhages
   2. bilateral retinal hemorrhages
   3. macular retinal folds

Consultative cause and manner of death

Cause of death: Acute meningitis complicated by sepsis, systemic inflammatory response syndrome, septic shock, and multiorgan system failure.

Manner of death: Natural.

Discussion

A thorough examination of the case file, to include all available investigative and medical information, failed to disclose any evidence to support the medical examiner's cause of death, "Complications of blunt force head injury." This infant was examined by a number of healthcare professionals and there was no evidence of external or internal injury (Figures 9.19 and 9.20). There were faint contusions as noted by the medical

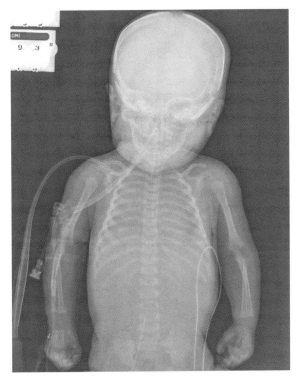

Figure 9.19 Anterior–posterior radiograph of the decedent with no evidence of skeletal trauma.

examiner consistent with medical manipulation and resuscitative efforts, but not blunt force injury, yet the case was certified as a homicide.

Meningitis is often difficult to diagnose in infants at autopsy because meningitis may not present as a purulent process. There were no gross stigmata of an acute inflammatory process on the surface of the decedent's cerebral cortex (Figures 9.21 and 9.22). When bacterial meningitis is suspected, the examining pathologist can microbiologically resolve it by performance of either a postmortem lumbar puncture for culture or using a bacterial culturette and taking a swab of the leptomeninges before the skull has been completely removed. In addition, occult inflammation can be resolved by stripping the leptomeninges from the surface of the brain, rolling them into a tissue cassette, and then examining them microscopically. At the request of the consulting neuropathologist, more brain tissue and leptomeninges were prepared and examined microscopically. The additional microscopic sections revealed infiltrates of acute inflammatory cells in the leptomeninges *not* associated with recent

83

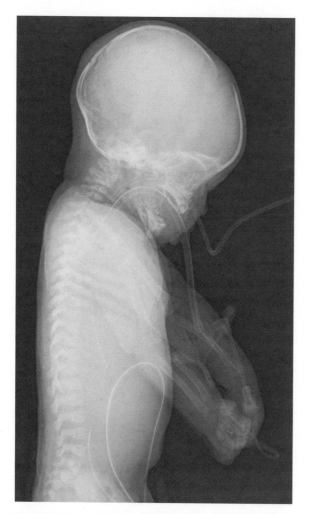

Figure 9.20 Lateral radiograph of the decedent with no evidence of skeletal trauma.

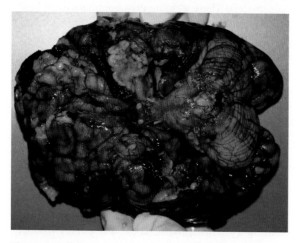

Figure 9.21 Inferior surface of the formalinized brain of the decedent with no evidence of purulent infectious process.

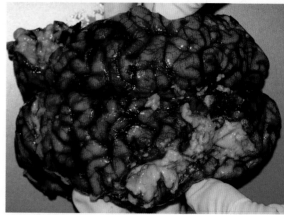

Figure 9.22 Superior surface of the formalinized brain of the decedent with no evidence of purulent infectious process.

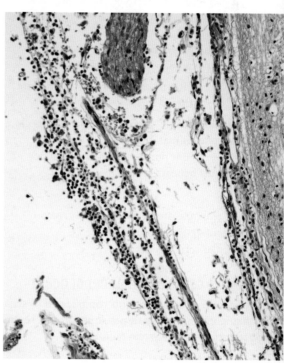

Figure 9.23 Medium power H&E micrograph of the leptomeninges demonstrating acute inflammatory infiltration.

hemorrhage (Figures 9.23 and 9.24). This confirmed the diagnosis of acute meningitis.

Infants often do not present with the same symptoms as older children and adults, and clinical–pathologic correlation is necessary, even when distracting findings such as subarachnoid and subdural hemorrhage are diagnosed in the complete absence

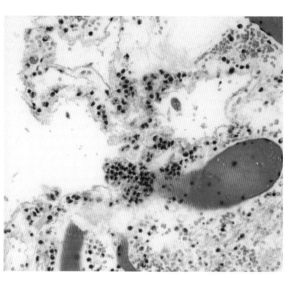

Figure 9.24 Medium power H&E micrograph of the leptomeninges demonstrating acute inflammatory infiltration.

of external trauma (Cohen and Scheimberg, 2009). Meningitis and traumatic head injury (accidental or intentionally inflicted) can present with similar symptoms, but the presence of fever and an elevated white blood cell count are key factors differentiating accidental or intentionally inflicted head injury from meningitis, because fever and an elevated white blood cell count are not associated with acute head injury.

The cause of death was acute meningitis complicated by sepsis, systemic inflammatory response syndrome, septic shock, and multiorgan system failure. As sequelae of her disease, the infant developed severe cerebral edema with increased intracranial pressure; diffuse, global hypoxic/ischemic encephalopathy; and a coagulopathy as part of systemic inflammatory response and multiorgan system failure.

The bilateral retinal and optic nerve sheath hemorrhages were, once again, due to the increased in intracranial pressure in response the infant's meningitis. If these hemorrhages were due to trauma, the trauma would have been evident anatomically. Again, retinal and/or optic nerve sheath hemorrhages do not independently indicate abusive head trauma. In the absence of anatomically demonstrable trauma, their presence must be further elucidated and correlated with other anatomic findings.

Few areas of forensic pathology have generated as much controversy as the reliability of retinal and optic

nerve sheath hemorrhages in diagnosing inflicted head injury. There is adequate literature supporting an increase in intracranial pressure (ICP) as a common cause of retinal and optic nerve sheath hemorrhages (Muller and Deck, 1974; Firsching et al., 2011). Terson syndrome, intra-ocular hemorrhage associated with subarachnoid hemorrhage, causes increased ICP resulting in retinal and optic nerve sheath hemorrhages (Mena et al., 2011), and numerous case reports have documented retinal and optic nerve sheath hemorrhage where accidental trauma resulted in cerebral edema and increased ICP (Lantz et al., 2004; Lantz and Stanton, 2006).

There is no pathognomonic pattern of retinal and optic nerve sheath hemorrhages representative of child abuse or any other disease process; therefore the presence of such hemorrhages in this particular case, at the exclusion of anatomically demonstrable trauma, is most consistent with increased ICP as published previously (Matshes, 2010). Retinal hemorrhages have been seen in newborn infants where there is documented increased ICP and absolutely no evidence of trauma, as well as with straining at stool or severe Valsalva maneuver, and even chest compressions during resuscitation. A recent paper in the journal *Pediatrics* describes retinal hemorrhages occurring in 15% of critically ill, historically non-abused children (Agrawal, 2012). In this paper the most severe hemorrhages were found in children who experienced severe accidental head trauma and coagulopathies.

In a young infant with fracture calluses, a set of differential diagnoses for the etiology of these fractures includes, but is not limited to: (1) birth trauma; (2) metabolic bone disease (e.g., vitamin D deficiency etc.); (3) non-accidental injury (NAI); (4) accidental trauma; and (5) osteogenesis imperfecta.

In the context of rib fractures in an infant, non-accidental injury must always be considered and investigated. When there are fractures present in different stages of healing, non-accidental injury should be strongly considered.

Comment by authors

The history and presenting symptoms must be always considered without reflexing to intentional or abusive injury as the cause of a child's demise. Although the absence of external and internal injury does not completely exclude intentional or abusive injury, when there are no apparent injuries, other causes must be considered and should guide and inform the anatomic and laboratory examination. Again, correlation of anatomic and laboratory findings with the history and/or investigative information is mandatory to avoid misinterpretation.

Death investigation system

As stated previously, the system of death investigation is charged by statute to determine cause and manner of death in cases within their jurisdiction(s). Cause of death is determined by death scene examination, autopsy, and laboratory analyses. But these determinations are a few facets of the profession. Other endeavors include interpretation of death scene findings in order to assist law enforcement in the commencement of their investigation, helping to identify and document wound patterns and to help to differentiate inflicted versus accidental injuries (in cases where this can be defensibly achieved), and the collection of evidence outside and inside the body as an adjunct to criminal investigations. The final goal of the system is not only to generate a concise autopsy report (or protocol), which stands as the final record of death (and sometimes evidence of life) for a person, but also to give medical and scientific assistance through all phases of investigation as well as providing expert witness testimony that is truly where the "rubber meets the road." The personnel involved in the death investigation system must convey the scene, investigatory, autopsy, and laboratory data clearly and concisely so that the judge and jury have full understanding of the scope of these cases without leading or permitting their opinions to stray far from the available objective data. Death investigators must interpret forensic scientific findings where and when they can in order to convey their importance in the case, yet this must be tempered with ambiguity where no interpretation can be made, and the distinction(s) must be made clear to the audience of the public forum. Forensic scientific findings must be interpreted with humility, in context, and never overinterpreted out of ignorance or self-importance (i.e., patterned injuries are "consistent with ..." or rarely "caused by ..."). Overinterpretation can be deadly to the case, and to a potentially innocent defendant. Finally, these practices and findings must be defensible from both a scientific and medical point of view – each and every time. These cases may go back to court over and over again following the initial trial, so practitioners must realize that their findings can be scrutinized by both criminal and civil elements of the legal system, and they must stand up each time, every time.

References

Agrawal S, Peters M J, Adams G G, Pierce C M. Prevalence of retinal hemorrhages in critically ill children. *Pediatrics*. 2012; 129e:e1388–96.

Board of Directors National Association of Medical Examiners. Inspection and accreditation checklist. Feb 2014.

Clark S C, Ernst M F, Haglund W D, Jentzen J M. *Medicolegal Death Investigator: A Systematic Training Program for the Professional Death Investigator*. Big Rapids, MI: Occupational Research and Assessment. 1996.

Cohen M C, Scheimberg I. Evidence of occurrence of intradural and subdural hemorrhage in the perinatal and neonatal period in the context of hypoxic ischemic encephalopathy: An observational study from two referral institutions in the United Kingdom. *Pediatric and Developmental Pathology*. 2009; 12:169–76.

Collins K A, Byard R W. (eds) *Forensic Pathology of Infancy and Childhood*. New York: Springer. 2014.

Desborough J P. The stress response to trauma and surgery. *British Journal of Anaesthesia*. 2000; 85:109–17.

Duhaime A C, Gennarelli T, Thibault L E, *et al*. The shaken baby syndrome: A clinical, pathological, and biomechanical study. *Journal of Neurosurgery*. 1987; 66:409–15.

Firsching R, Muller C, Pauli S U. Noninvasive assessment of intracranial pressure with venous ophthalmodynamometry. *Neurosurgery*. 2011; 115:371–4.

Geddes J F, Hackenshaw A K, Vowles G H, Nickols C D, Whitwell H L. Neuropathology of inflicted head injury in children I. Patterns of injury. *Brain*. 2001; 124:1290–8.

Lantz P E, Sinal S H, Stanton C A, Weaver R G, Jr. Perimacular retinal folds from childhood head trauma. *British Medical Journal*. 2004; 328:754–6.

Lantz P E, Stanton C A. Postmortem detection and evaluation of retinal hemorrhages. Presented at the *American Academy of Forensic Sciences Annual Meeting*, Seattle, WA. Feb 2006.

Matshes E. Retinal and optic nerve sheath hemorrhages are not pathognomonic of abusive head injury. *American Academy of Forensic Sciences Annual Meeting*. 2010; 272.

Matshes E W, Evans R M, Pinckard J K, Joseph J T, Lew E O. Shaken infants die of neck trauma, not brain trauma. *Academic Forensic Pathology*. 2011; 1(1):82–91.

Mena O J, Paul I, Richard R R. Ocular findings in raised intracranial pressure: A case of Terson syndrome in a 7-month-old infant. *American Journal of Forensic Medicine and Pathology*. 2011; 32(1):55–7.

Muller P J, Deck J H N. Intraocular and optic nerve sheath hemorrhage in cases of sudden intracranial hypertension. *Journal of Neurosurgery*. 1974; 41:160–6.

NAME. Forensic autopsy performance standards. National Association of Medical Examiners. 2015, p. 9. www.fameonline.org/images/fame_files/Standards/2015_NAME_Forensic_Autopsy_Performance_Standards.pdf [Accessed Feb 25, 2016].

National Medicolegal Review Panel. Death Investigation: A Guide for the Scene Investigator. U.S. Department of Justice Office of Justice Programs Research Report. 1999.

Pathak A, Dutta S, Marwaha N, *et al*. Change in tissue thromboplastin content of brain following trauma. *Neurology India*. 2005; 53:178–82.

Peterson G F, Clark S C. *Forensic Autopsy Performance Standards*. National Association of Medical Examiners, 2012.

Prange M T, Coats B, Duhaime A C, Margulies S S. Anthropomorphic simulations of falls, shakes, and inflected impacts in infants. *Journal of Neurosurgery*. 2003; 99:143–50.

Robinson R M, Trelka D P. Forensic scene investigation. *eMedicine*. 2011; Medscape.com.

Technical Working Group on Crime Scene Investigation. Crime scene investigation: A guide for law enforcement. U.S. Department of Justice Office of Justice Programs Research Report. 2000.

Index